NEUROLOGY - LABORATORY AND CLINICAL
RESEARCH DEVELOPMENTS

NEUROFIBROMATOSIS

DIAGNOSIS, MANAGEMENT AND CLINICAL OUTCOMES

NEUROLOGY - LABORATORY AND CLINICAL RESEARCH DEVELOPMENTS

Additional books in this series can be found on Nova's website
under the Series tab.

Additional E-books in this series can be found on Nova's website
under the E-book tab.

NEUROLOGY - LABORATORY AND CLINICAL
RESEARCH DEVELOPMENTS

NEUROFIBROMATOSIS

DIAGNOSIS, MANAGEMENT AND CLINICAL OUTCOMES

WALTER ROMAINE
EDITOR

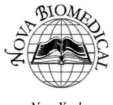

New York

Library of Congress Cataloging-in-Publication Data

ISBN: 978-1-63463-229-4

Library of Congress Control Number: 2014952258

Published by Nova Science Publishers, Inc. † New York

CONTENTS

PREFACE

Neurofibromatosis Type 1 (NF1) is a hereditary neurocutaneous tumor disorder that owes many of its most common features to abnormalities in neural crest-derived cells. NF1 may cause dysplasia in various tissues, even in some tissues that are non-neural crest-derived (e.g. bone). While common manifestations of NF1 include café-au-lait spots and neurofibromas, vasculopathies are less common yet noteworthy complications of NF1. NF1 vasculopathies can involve vessels supplying various organs. Cerebrovascular abnormalities associated with NF1 have been sporadically described in the literature; these conditions are of interest due to the incomplete understanding of their pathogenesis and genetics. This book discusses the diagnosis, managements and clinical outcomes for neurofibromatosis.

Chapter 1 - Neurofibromatosis type 1 (NF-1) is a relatively rare autosomal dominant neurocutaneous genetic disorder, affecting 1 in 3000 – 4000 individuals, with the cardinal features of café au lait macules, benign neurofibromas, and iris hamartomas. Vascular abnormalities, mostly in the form of aneurysms or stenoses, affect medium and large vessels and are recognized manifestations of NF-1; these vascular lesions have been reported to occur in 0.41% – 6.4% of patients. Cervical pseudoaneurysms associated with NF-1 are rare. Although rare, these aneurysms often present with life-threatening spontaneous rupture or neurological complications. The pathogenesis and natural history of these vascular lesions remain unknown. The present study was performed to review the spectrum, management, and clinical outcome of patients with extracranial cervical pseudoaneurysm associated with NF-1. Ten cases of extracranial internal carotid artery, including the authors' case, a case of common carotid artery, 6 cases of external carotid artery, and 21 cases of extracranial vertebral artery pseudoaneurysms in patients with NF-1 have been reported in the English and Japanese literature between 1967 and 2014. The mean age at the time of diagnosis was 43.2 years (range, 1 – 66 years). Twelve patients were men and 25 were women. Seven patients were incidental cases. In the remaining 31 cases, the symptoms were ruptured pseudoaneurysm (18 cases), expanding mass or growth (6 cases), and radiculopathy (5 cases). The treatments were surgery in 9 cases, endovascular treatment in 19 cases, and the remaining 10 cases received conservative treatment or were untreated. Most cases were associated with a favorable recovery, with recovery from the initial symptoms. Mortality was mostly associated with untreated cases or death from concomitant ruptured abdominal aortic aneurysm. Surgical repair and vessel reconstruction are limited by arterial fragility in patients with NF-1. An endovascular approach, such as stenting and coil embolization, is preferable in high-risk patients.

Chapter 2 - Neurofibromatosis type 1 (NF1), also known as von Recklinghausen disease, is a common autosomal dominant genetic disorder affecting approximately 1 in 3000 individuals worldwide. NF1 results from heritable or spontaneous mutations of the NF1 tumor suppressor gene, encoding the protein neurofibromin, which functions to negatively regulate Ras-activity. Although neurofibromas are considered the hallmark feature of NF1, up to 70 percent of NF1 patients develop both generalized and focal osseous defects including short stature, kyphoscoliosis, osteopenia/osteoporosis, fractures, and pseudarthrosis (fracture non-union). While defective osteoblast bone anabolism has been implicated as a central factor in the pathogenesis of NF1 associated skeletal deficits, recent data suggests that NF1 (Nf1) haploinsufficiency within the hematopoietic compartment, particularly in osteoclasts and myeloid progenitors, plays a pivotal role in engendering NF1 osseous manifestations. In this chapter, the authors review the latest data from clinical studies and murine models demonstrating a requirement for hematopoietic derived NF1 (Nf1) haploinsufficient osteoclasts and their progenitors in the pathogenesis of multiple NF1 skeletal deficits.

Chapter 3 - Neurofibromatosis Type 1 (NF1) is a hereditary neurocutaneous tumor disorder that owes many of its most common features to abnormalities in neural crest-derived cells. NF1 may cause dysplasia in various tissues, even in some tissues that are non-neural crest-derived (e.g. bone). While common manifestations of NF1 include café-au-lait spots and neurofibromas, vasculopathies are less common yet noteworthy complications of NF1. NF1 vasculopathies can involve vessels supplying various organs.

Cerebrovascular abnormalities associated with NF1 have been sporadically described in the literature; these conditions are of interest due to the incomplete understanding of their pathogenesis and genetics.

NF1 is associated with a diverse set of cerebrovascular complications including stenosis/occlusive disease, aneurysm, arteriovenous malformations, Moya Moya disease, arteriovenous fistulas, spontaneous vascular rupture, and arteries compressed or invaded by neural tumors. The most common cerebrovascular abnormality in NF1 patients is occlusion or stenosis of the cerebral arteries. In this chapter, the authors describe the cerebrovascular complications of NF1 focusing on the pathology of the aforementioned subtypes, pathogenesis, clinical features, outcomes, proposed therapies and genetics.

Chapter 4 - Neurofibromatosis type 1 (NF1) affects 1 in 3,500 people and is one of the most common genetic disorders with a predisposition to malignancy. NF1 is caused by autosomal dominant mutations in the *NF1* tumor suppressor gene, which encodes neurofibromin, a negative regulator of Ras-activity. Cutaneous and plexiform neurofibromas, the hallmark tumors of NF1, are heterogeneous neoplasms composed of tumorigenic Schwann cells and a complex microenvironment, including mast cells, fibroblasts, and blood vessels. Emerging evidence indicates a pivotal role for interactions between Schwann cells, surrounding stroma, and hematopoietic constituents of the tumor microenvironment in promoting neurofibroma genesis. In NF1 mouse models, tumorigenic *Nf1* nullizygous Schwan cells secrete supraphysiologic levels of stem cell factor (SCF), co-opting *Nf1* haploinsufficient mast cells to infiltrate the tumor microenvironment. In turn, activated $Nf1^{+/-}$ mast cells secrete multiple inflammatory effectors which potentiate fibroblast proliferation, collagen deposition and angiogenesis, thereby creating a viscous cycle perpetuating neurofibroma maintenance and expansion. Experimental evidence from NF1 murine models indicates that either genetic or pharmacologic inhibition of SCF/c-kit dependent mast cell recruitment /activation is sufficient to treat neurofibromas in the NF1 murine model. A recent phase 2 clinical trial using Gleevec, which targets multi-tyrosine kinases including c-kit, provided the first evidence of an effective therapy for the treatment of plexiform neurofibromas. This chapter will review current clinical and animal model data delineating the role of the tumor microenvironment in neurofibroma pathogenesis and therapy.

In: Neurofibromatosis
Editor: Walter Romaine

ISBN: 978-1-63463-229-4
© 2015 Nova Science Publishers, Inc.

Chapter 1

CERVICAL PSEUDOANEURYSM ASSOCIATED WITH NEUROFIBROMATOSIS TYPE 1

Osamu Hamasaki[*1] *and Kaoru Kurisu*[2]

[1]Department of Neurosurgery,
Shimane Prefectural Central Hospital, Izumo, Japan
[2]Department of Neurosurgery,
Hiroshima University Graduate School of Biomedical and Health Sciences,
Hiroshima, Japan

ABSTRACT

Neurofibromatosis type 1 (NF-1) is a relatively rare autosomal dominant neurocutaneous genetic disorder, affecting 1 in 3000 – 4000 individuals, with the cardinal features of café au lait macules, benign neurofibromas, and iris hamartomas. Vascular abnormalities, mostly in the form of aneurysms or stenoses, affect medium and large vessels and are recognized manifestations of NF-1; these vascular lesions have been reported to occur in 0.41%–6.4% of patients. Cervical pseudoaneurysms associated with NF-1 are rare. Although rare, these aneurysms often present with life-threatening spontaneous rupture or neurological complications. The pathogenesis and natural history of these vascular lesions remain unknown. The present study was performed to review the

[*] Corresponding author: Osamu Hamasaki, M.D., Department of Neurosurgery, Shimane Prefectural Central Hospital, 4-1-1 Himebara, Izumo, Shimane 693-8555, Japan. TEL: +81-853-22-5111. Fax: +81-853-21-2975. E-mail address: ohamasa@orange.ocn.ne.jp.

spectrum, management, and clinical outcome of patients with extracranial cervical pseudoaneurysm associated with NF-1. Ten cases of extracranial internal carotid artery, including our case, a case of common carotid artery, 6 cases of external carotid artery, and 21 cases of extracranial vertebral artery pseudoaneurysms in patients with NF-1 have been reported in the English and Japanese literature between 1967 and 2014. The mean age at the time of diagnosis was 43.2 years (range, 1 – 66 years). Twelve patients were men and 25 were women. Seven patients were incidental cases. In the remaining 31 cases, the symptoms were ruptured pseudoaneurysm (18 cases), expanding mass or growth (6 cases), and radiculopathy (5 cases). The treatments were surgery in 9 cases, endovascular treatment in 19 cases, and the remaining 10 cases received conservative treatment or were untreated. Most cases were associated with a favorable recovery, with recovery from the initial symptoms. Mortality was mostly associated with untreated cases or death from concomitant ruptured abdominal aortic aneurysm. Surgical repair and vessel reconstruction are limited by arterial fragility in patients with NF-1. An endovascular approach, such as stenting and coil embolization, is preferable in high-risk patients.

Keyword: Neurofibromatosis type 1, cervical, pseudoaneurysm, fragility, surgery, endovascular treatment

INTRODUCTION

Neurofibromatosis type 1 (NF-1) is a relatively rare autosomal dominant neurocutaneous genetic disorder, affecting one in 3000 – 4000 individuals, with the cardinal features of café au lait macules, benign neurofibromas, and iris hamartomas [26]. Vascular abnormalities, mostly in the form of aneurysms or stenosis, affect medium and large vessels, and are recognized manifestations of NF-1; these vascular lesions have been reported to occur in 0.41%–6.4% of patients [28]. The renal artery is most frequently involved, but abdominal aortic coarctation, internal carotid artery (ICA) aneurysms, and vertebral arteriovenous malformations have also been reported. Cervical pseudoaneurysms associated with NF-1 are rare. Although rare, these aneurysms often present with life-threatening spontaneous rupture or neurological complications. The pathogenesis and natural history of these vascular lesions remain unknown. The present study was performed to review the pertinent literature regarding patients with extracranial cervical pseudoaneurysm associated with NF-1.

LITTERATURE REVIEW

We reviewed cases of cervical pseudoaneurysm in patients with NF-1 reported in the English and Japanese literature between 1967 and 2014 (Table 1) [1, 2, 6, 7, 9, 11-18, 20-25, 27-33, 36, 39, 41, 42, 44-46, 47, 49]. As there have been no prospective studies, all retrospective articles and case reports were included. Arterial lesions were located in the extracranial ICA in 10 cases, including our case, in the common carotid artery (CCA) in 1 case, the external carotid artery (ECA) in 6 cases, and the extracranial vertebral artery (VA) in 21 cases. The mean age at the time of diagnosis was 43.2 years (range, 1–66 years). Twelve patients were men and 25 were women. Seven patients were incidental cases. In the remaining 31 cases, the symptoms were ruptured pseudoaneurysm (18 cases), expanding mass or growth (6 cases), and radiculopathy (5 cases). The treatments were surgery in 9 cases, endovascular treatment in 19 cases, and the other 10 cases received conservative treatment or were untreated. Most cases were associated with a favorable recovery, with recovery from initial the symptoms. Mortality was mostly associated with untreated cases or death from concomitant ruptured abdominal aortic aneurysm. Surgical repair and vessel reconstruction are limited by arterial fragility in patients with NF-1.

DISCUSSION

NF-1 is caused by mutations of the *NF-1* gene located on chromosome 17q11.2 [48]. The protein product of the NF-1 gene is neurofibromin. Thus, neurofibromin deficiency may be linked to NF-1 vasculopathy. The main hypothesis proposed by Riccardi [34] is that the vasculopathy is caused by alteration of the normal process of vascular maintenance and repair regulated by neurofibromin. Vascular abnormalities (e.g., arterial stenoses and aneurysms) in patients with NF-1 occur via a dynamic process of cellular proliferation, degeneration, healing, smooth muscle loss, and fibrosis [8]. Vascular endothelial and smooth muscle cells express neurofibromin. The prevalence of vascular abnormalities associated with NF-1 is 0.4%–6.4% [28]. Most patients with NF-1-related vascular abnormalities are asymptomatic, but multiple vessels are usually involved.

Table 1. Summary of patients with extracranial cervical pseudoaneurysm associated with Neurofibromatosis type 1

Series [ref. no.]	Age/Sex	Side	Artery	Symptom	Ruptured	Treatment	Outcome
Kamiyama et al. 1985 [18]	56/F	Right	ICA	Asymptomatic	no	Conservative	Alive
Frank et al. 1989 [7]	18/M	Right	ICA	Asymptomatic	no	Conservative	Alive
Shibuya et al. 1994 [36]	33/F	Left	ICA	Spontaneous rupture	yes	Surgery, not stopped bleeding	Dead
Smith et al. 2000 [42]	28/F	Left	ICA	Spontaneous rupture	yes	Stent graft	Alive
Kobayashi et al. 2006 [20]	66/M	Left	ICA	Spontaneous rupture	yes	Surgical trapping with bypass	Dead
Ku et al. 2008 [21]	28/F	Bilateral	ICA	Stroke and rupture	yes	Left sacrifice, right endovascular trapping	Alive
Onkendi et al. 2010 [30]	42/F	Right	ICA	Expanding mass	no	Surgery (excism and bypass)	Alive
You et al. 2011 [49]	17/M	Bilateral	ICA	Asymptomatic	no	Conservative	Alive
Moratti et al. 2012 [24]	48/F	Right	ICA	Expanding mass	no	Endovascular trapping using DB, coil, liquid	Alive
Hamasaki et al. 2014 [9]	66/F	Right	ICA	Aneurysm growth (ITA aneurysm rupture)	no	Stenting and coil embolization	Alive
Pearce 1967 [31]	36/F	Left	CCA	Expanding mass	no	Untreated (autopsy)	no follow
Pearce 1967 [31]	40/F	Right	ECA	Expanding mass	no	Untreated (autopsy)	no follow
Abe et al. 1998 [1]	53/F	Right	ECA	Spontaneous rupture	yes	Surgical ligation	Alive
Smith et al. 2000 [42]	28/F	Left	ECA	Asymptomatic (ICA aneurysm rupture)	no	Coil embolization	Alive
Takeda et al. 2002 [45]	52/M	Right	ECA	Spontaneous rupture	yes	Coil embolization	Dead
Takeda et al. 2002 [45]	60/F	Left	ECA	Spontaneous rupture	yes	Coil embolization	Alive
Takeda et al. 2010 [44]	43/M	Left	ECA	Spontaneous rupture	yes	Coil embolization	Alive
Schubiger et al. 1978 [41]	50/M	Left	VA	Radiculopathy	no	Surgery	Alive
Pentecost et al. 1981 [32]	1/F	Left	VA	Limited cervical movement	no	Conservative (surgery of other aneurysm)	Alive

Series [ref. no.]	Age/Sex	Side	Artery	Symptom	Ruptured	Treatment	Outcome
Detwiler et al. 1987 [6]	52/F	Left	VA	Radiculopathy	no	Proximal occlusion using DB	Alive
Negoro et al. 1990 [27]	47/M	Left	VA	Spontaneous rupture	yes	Proximal occlusion using DB	Alive
Ueda et al. 1990 [46]	51/M	Left	VA	Asymptomatic (intracranial AN rupture)	no	Conservative (surgery of other aneurysm)	Alive
Schievink et al. 1991 [39]	43/F	Left	VA	Asymptomatic	no	Conservative	Alive
Muhonen et al. 1991 [25]	52/F	Left	VA	Expanding mass	no	Occlusion using DB	Alive
Ohkata et al. 1994 [29]	48/F	Left	VA	Radiculopathy	no	Surgery	Alive
Horsley et al. 1997 [17]	56/F	Left	VA	Spontaneous rupture	yes	Occlusion using DB	Alive
Hoffmann et al. 1998 [15]	59/M	Right	VA	Asymptomatic	no	Conservative	Alive
Magara et al. 1998 [22]	28/M	Left	VA	Spontaneous rupture	yes	Surgery	Alive
Ushikoshi et al. 1999 [47]	40/F	Left	VA	Spontaneous rupture	yes	Proximal occlusion using DB	Alive
Miyazaki et al. 2004 [23]	52/F	Left	VA	Spontaneous rupture	yes	Surgery following balloon occlusion	Dead
Arai et al. 2007 [2]	38/M	Left	VA	Spontaneous rupture	yes	Untreated	Dead
Hieda et al. 2007 [11]	36/F	Left	VA	Spontaneous rupture	yes	Coil and Liquid embolization	Alive
Oderich et al. 2007 [28]	43/F	Left	VA	Spontaneous rupture	yes	Surgery (subclavian artery ligation with bypass)	Alive
Hiramatsu et al. 2007 [14]	67/M	Left	VA	dizziness	no	Coil embolization	Alive
Peyre et al. 2007 [33]	18/F	Right	VA	Radiculopathy	no	Coil embolization	Alive
Horie et al. 2008 [16]	30/F	Left	VA	Radiculopathy	no	Coil embolization and DB placement	Alive
Higa et al. 2010 [12]	60/F	Left	VA	Spontaneous rupture	yes	Coil embolization	Alive
Hiramatsu et al. 2012 [13]	40/F	Right	VA	Spontaneous rupture	yes	Coil embolization	Alive

CCA common carotid artery, DB detachable balloon, ECA external carotid artery, F female, ICA internal carotid artery, ITA internal thoracic artery, M male , VA vertebral artery.

The term NF-1 vasculopathy has been coined to describe vascular abnormalities that involve medium-, large-, and small-sized arteries and veins in patients with NF-1 [10, 28]. The most common clinical presentation is difficult to control hypertension associated with renal artery stenosis in childhood [28, 42].

The most common cause of death in patients with NF-1 is malignancy; however, in patients younger than 40, vascular disease and hypertension are the second leading causes of death [28, 35]. Cerebrovascular abnormalities include occlusion of major intracranial vessels, arteriovenous malformations, and intracranial aneurysms. Schievink et al. [40] detected incidental intracranial aneurysms in two (5%) of 39 patients with NF-1 who were hospitalized for other reasons, suggesting that patients with NF-1 are at increased risk of developing intracranial aneurysm as a vascular manifestation of NF-1. On the other hand, to study the relationship between NF-1 and intracranial aneurysms, Conway et al. [5] analyzed all intracranial autopsies of NF-1 patients performed at their institution and analyzed all cases of intracranial aneurysm at their institution in an attempt to identify patients with NF-1. They concluded that there is a lack of evidence for any association between NF-1 and intracranial aneurysms. Oderich et al. [28] reviewed 76 vascular abnormalities in 31 patients with NF-1. Arterial lesions were located in the aorta ($n = 17$ lesions), renal artery ($n = 12$), mesenteric artery ($n = 12$), carotid-vertebral artery ($n = 10$), intracerebral artery ($n = 4$), subclavian-axillary artery ($n = 3$), and iliofemoral artery ($n = 3$). ICA aneurysms accounted for only 4 (5.2%) of 76 vascular abnormalities. Furthermore, Oderich et al. [28] reviewed 237 patients with NF-1, with 320 vascular abnormalities, reported in the English literature. Renal artery lesions were the most common (41%) and were more often stenotic than aneurysmal. Lesions affecting the carotid, vertebral, or cerebral artery (19% of patients) were commonly aneurysms. In addition, the authors reviewed 30 ICA aneurysms in 29 patients with NF-1 reported in the English literature between 1957 and 2005. Epidemiologically, it is unclear whether intracranial or cervical aneurysm associated with NF-1 represents the largest number of cases, but it is thought that cervical lesions belong to a larger group of symptomatic aneurysms. ICA aneurysms in patients with NF-1 are often associated with spontaneous rupture and bleeding, with pregnancy reported as a strong predisposing factor. Sobata et al. [43] reported a case of a ruptured intracranial ICA aneurysm in a 28-year-old woman that occurred immediately after delivery. Shibuya et al. [36] reported a case of ruptured extracranial ICA aneurysm in a 33-year-old woman, 9 days postpartum. Smith et al. [42] also reported a case of a ruptured extracranial ICA aneurysm in a 28-year-old woman, 10 days postpartum.

With regard to the treatment of cervical pseudoaneurysm in extracranial ICA and CCA, it is possible that sacrifice of the affected artery is unsuitable. Although most patients with NF-1-associated vascular lesions are asymptomatic, treatment is usually recommended in cases of carotid artery aneurysms with symptoms such as cerebral ischemia, mass effect, or rupture. The treatment of cervical pseudoaneurysm in extracranial ICA and CCA included sacrifice or trapping in 3 cases, surgical repair in 1 case, stent graft in 1 case, and stenting and coil embolization in 1 case (Table 1). Surgical repair is aggressive and complex, and vessel reconstruction is limited by arterial fragility in patients with NF-1 [19]. The operative exposure is judged to be difficult for lesions with extension of the aneurysm to the distal ICA. In addition, negative effects of parent vessel sacrifice include the increased risk of hemodynamic impairment in patients with a single carotid artery as well as the risk of formation of flow-related de novo aneurysms in other mainly contralateral arteries that will now have increased flow. Endovascular repair with intraluminal stent grafting have been performed successfully in cases where access for distal arterial control with operative exposure is considered challenging and unsafe. However, unfavorable anatomy of the ICA, including severe kink, loop, or tortuosity or the ICA proximal to the aneurysm, makes the use of stent grafts difficult and may increase the risk of complications with an endovascular approach. Smith et al. [42] reported a case of successful repair, and concluded that although this mode of repair is feasible, but difficult, it is a better option than open repair in cases with difficult distal exposure of the involved vessels. In contrast, a combination of endovascular stenting and coil embolization to prevent bleeding and re-establish blood flow has been reported in patients with ECA and ICA aneurysm [4]. However, our patient is the first reported example of successful endovascular stenting and coil embolization for extracranial ICA pseudoaneurysm in patients with NF-1 [9]. Self-expanding stents are used to treat intracranial ICA aneurysms. Furthermore, the combination of endovascular stenting and coil embolization has been reported in patients with intracranial ICA pseudoaneurysm [4]. Flexible stents may compress the pseudoaneurysm inflow tract, inducing stasis, facilitating intraaneurysmal thrombosis; the thrombosis acts as an endoluminal scaffold to prevent coil herniation into the parent artery, allowing tight packing of even a wide-necked and irregularly shaped aneurysm and serving as a matrix for endothelial growth. Assali et al. [3] evaluated the potential of using flexible self-expanding uncovered stents with or without coiling to treat extracranial internal carotid, subclavian, and other peripheral artery posttraumatic pseudoaneurysms. They concluded that uncovered endovascular flexible self-expanding stent placement with trans-stent coil embolization of the pseudoaneurysm cavity is a promising technique for treating such vascular diseases using minimally invasive methods while preserving the patency of the vessel and side branches. Sakamoto et al. [37] successfully performed endovascular stenting and coil embolization for ruptured subclavian artery pseudoaneurysms associated with NF-1. Stent placement revealed the risks of both thromboembolism and stent occlusion requiring meticulous anti-thromboembolic treatment. In our experience, endovascular stenting and coil embolization for extracranial ICA aneurysm associated with NF-1 was considered safe and effective. More recently, stenting techniques using flow diverters have been proposed for the treatment of giant and large aneurysms. Flow diverters appear to be promising tools even though the risks and outcomes of such treatment are still not well known, especially in cases with known underlying disease, such as NF-1.

On the other hand, treatment of cervical pseudoaneurysm in VA and ECA involved sacrifice of the affected artery and included trapping using coil embolization in 10 cases, surgical ligation or bypass in 6 cases, and proximal occlusion using detachable balloons in 4 cases (Table 1). Most aneurysms were of the fusiform type, so surgical trapping and removal of the aneurysm, or endovascular trapping with coils and/or detachable balloons were indicated. If only proximal occlusion of the parent artery is performed, the aneurysm may not disappear and will be recanalized by blood flow from the opposite VA and other collateral vessels. Therefore, endovascular trapping of the distal parent artery is thought to be a better treatment modality. Direct surgery was selected in earlier cases, whereas endovascular treatment was chosen in more recent cases. Endovascular treatment has the advantage of being minimally invasive and with short operation duration, particularly for ruptured aneurysms.

Most cases were associated with a favorable recovery, with recovery from the initial symptoms. Mortality was mostly associated with untreated cases or death from concomitant ruptured abdominal aortic aneurysm. As the prognosis of patients with ruptured aneurysms is extremely poor, unruptured aneurysms should be treated before rupture. Surgical repair and vessel reconstruction are limited by arterial fragility in patients with NF-1 [19]. An endovascular approach, such as stenting and coil embolization, is preferable especially in high-risk patients. As our study involved retrospective data acquisition, a prospective study with a more rigorous technical and follow-up strategy is warranted.

CONCLUSION

We have reviewed cervical pseudoaneurysms in patients with NF-1 reported in the English and Japanese literature between 1967 and 2014. Ten cases of extracranial ICA, including our case, 1 case of CCA, 6 cases of ECA, and 21 cases of extracranial VA pseudoaneurysms in patients with NF-1 have been reported. The treatments were surgery in 9 cases, endovascular treatment in 19 cases, and the remaining 10 cases received conservative treatment or were untreated. Most cases were associated with favorable recovery, with recovery from the initial symptoms. Mortality was mostly associated with untreated cases or death from concomitant ruptured abdominal aortic aneurysm. Surgical repair and vessel reconstruction are limited by arterial fragility in patients with NF-1. An endovascular approach, such as stenting and coil embolization, is preferable especially in high-risk patients.

REFERENCES

[1]   Abe, S., Yatsuduka, H., Soutsu, M., Sakai, H., Nakamura, N. (1988). A case of von Recklinghausen disease leading to massive subcutaneous bleeding in the neck. *Surgical diagnosis & treatment* 30, 673-676.

[2]   Arai, K., Sanada, J., Kurozumi, A., Watanabe, T., Matsui, O. (2007). Spontaneous hemothorax in neurofibromatosis treated with percutaneous embolization. *Cardiovasc Intervent Radiol* 30, 477-479.

[3]   Assali, AR., Sdringola, S., Moustapha, A., Rihner, M., Denktas, AE., Lefkowitz, MA., Campbell, M., Smalling, RW. (2001). Endovascular repair of traumatic pseudo-aneurysm by uncover self-expandable stenting with or without trans-stent coiling of the aneurysm cavity. *Catheter Cardiovasc Interv* 53, 253-258.

[4]   Bush, RL., Lin, PH., Dodson, TF., Dion, JE., Lumsden, AB. (2001). Endoluminal stent placement and coil embolization for the management of carotid artery pseudo-aneurysms. *J Endovasc Ther* 8, 53-61.

[5]   Conway, JE., Hutchins, GM., Tamargo, RJ. (2001). Lack of evidence for an association between neurofibromatosis type I and intracranial

aneurysms: autopsy study and review of the literature. *Stroke* 32, 2481-2485.

[6] Detwiler, K., Godersky, JC., Gentry, L. (1987). Pseudoaneurysm of the extracranial vertebral artery. *Case report. J Neurosurg* 67, 935-939.

[7] Frank, E., Brown, BM., Wilson, DF. (1989). Asymptomatic fusiform aneurysm of the petrous carotid artery in a patient with von Recklinghausen's Neurofibromatosis. *Surg Neurol* 32,75-78.

[8] Friedman, JM., Arbiser, J., Epstein, JA., Gutmann, DH., Huot, SJ., Lin, AE., Mcmanus, B., Krof, BR. (2002). Cardiovascular disease in Neurofibromatosis 1: report of the NF1 Cardiovascular Task Force. *Genet Med* 4, 105-111.

[9] Hamasaki, O., Ikawa, F., Hidaka, T., Kurokawa, Y., Yonezawa, U. (2014). Extracranial internal carotid artery pseudoaneurysm associated with neurofibromatosis type 1 treated with endovascular stenting and coil embolization. *Vasc Endovascular Surg* 48, 176-179.

[10] Hamilton, SJ. Friedman, JM. (2000). Insights into the pathogenesis of Neurofibromatosis 1 vasculopathy. *Clin Genet* 58, 341-344.

[11] Hieda, M., Toyota, N., Kakizawa, H., Hirai, N., Tachikake, T., Yahiro, Y., Iwasaki, Y., Horiguchi, J., Ito, K. (2007). Endovascular therapy for massive haemothorax caused by ruptured extracranial vertebral artery aneurysm with neurofibromatosis Type 1. *Br J Radiol.* 80, e81-84.

[12] Higa, G., Pacanowski, JP Jr., Jeck, DT., Goshima, KR., León, LR Jr. (2010). Vertebral artery aneurysms and cervical arteriovenous fistulae in patients with neurofibromatosis 1. *Vascular* 18, 166-177.

[13] Hiramatsu, H., Matsui, S., Yamashita, S., Kamiya, M., Yamashita, T., Akai, K., Watanabe, K., Namba, H. (2012). Ruptured extracranial vertebral artery aneurysm associated with neurofibromatosis type 1. Case report. *Neurol Med Chir* (Tokyo) 52, 446-449.

[14] Hiramatsu, H., Negoro, M., Hayakawa, M., Sadatou, A., Irie, K., Uemura, A., Kanno, T., Sano, K. (2007). Extracranial vertebral artery aneurysm associated with neurofibromatosis type 1. A case report. *Interv Neuroradiol* 15, 90-93.

[15] Hoffmann, KT., Hosten, N., Liebig, T., Schwarz, K., Felix, R. (1998). Giant aneurysm of the vertebral artery in neurofibromatosis type 1: report of a case and review of the literature. *Neuroradiology* 40, 245-248.

[16] Horie, N., Morikawa, M., Kitagawa, N., Nakamoto, M., Nagata, I. (2008). Successful endovascular occlusion of an aneurysm of the

cervical vertebral artery associated with neurofibromatosis-1. *Acta Neurochir* (Wien) 150, 847-848.

[17] Horsley, M., Taylor, TK., Sorby, WA. (1997). Traction-induced rupture of an extracranial vertebral artery aneurysm associated with neurofibromatosis. A case report. *Spine* 22, 225-227.

[18] Kamiyama, K., Endo, S., Horie, Y., Koshu, K., Takaku, A. (1985). Neurofibromatosis associated with intra- and extracranial aneurysms and extracranial vertebral arteriovenous fistula. *No Shinkei Geka* 13, 875-880.

[19] Kim, SJ., Kim, CW., Kim, S., Lee, TH., Kim, KI., Moon, TY., Chung, SW. (2005). Endovascular treatment of a ruptured internal thoracic aretery pseudo-aneurysm presenting as a massive haemothorax in a patient with type I Neurofibromatosis. *Caridovasc Intervent Radiol* 28, 818-821.

[20] Kobayashi, Y., Oshihma, O., Fujita, T., Takahashi, M., Harabuchi Y. (2006). A case of extracranial internal carotid artery aneurysm with Recklinghausen's disease. *Practica Oto-Rhino-Laryngologica* 99, 881-887.

[21] Ku, YK., Chen, HW., Chen, HW., Fu, CJ., Chin, SC., Liu, YC. (2008). Giant extracranial aneurysms of both internal carotid arteries with aberrant jugular veins in a patient with Neurofibromatosis type 1. *Am J Neuroradiol* 29, 1750-1752.

[22] Magara, T., Onoe, M., Yamamoto, Y., Kawakami, K., Hirai, T., Matsumoto, M. (1998). Massive mediastinal bleeding due to spontaneous rupture of the vertebral artery in von Recklinghausen disease. *Jpn J Thorac Cardiovasc Surg* 46, 906-909.

[23] Miyazaki, T., Ohta, F., Daisu, M., Hoshii, Y. (2004). Extracranial vertebral artery aneurysm ruptured into the thoracic cavity with neurofibromatosis type 1: case report. *Neurosurgery* 54, 1517-1520.

[24] Moratti, C., Andersson, T. (2012). Giant extracranial aneurysm of the internal carotid artery in neurofibromatosis type 1. A case report and review of the literature. *Interv Neuroradiol* 18, 341-347.

[25] Muhonen, MG., Godersky, JC., VanGilder, JC. (1991). Cerebral aneurysms associated with neurofibromatosis. Surg Neurol 36, 470-5.

[26] National Institutes of health Consensus Development Conference. (1988). Neurofibromatosis: conference statement. *Arch Neurol* 45, 575-578.

[27] Negoro, M., Nakaya, T., Terashima, K., Sugita, K. (1990). Extracranial vertebral artery aneurysm with neurofibromatosis. Endovascular treatment by detachable balloon. *Neuroradiology* 31, 533-536.

[28] Oderich, GS., Sullivan, TM., Bower, TC., Gloviczki, P., Miller, DV., Babovic-Vuksanovic, D., Macedo, TA., Stanson, A. (2007). Vascular abnormalities in patients with Neurofibromatosis syndrome type I: clinical spectrum, management, and results. *J Vasc Surg* 46, 475-484.

[29] Ohkata, N., Ikota, T., Tashiro, T., Okamoto, K. (1994). A case of multiple extracranial vertebral artery aneurysms associated with neurofibromatosis. *No Shinkei Geka* 22, 637-641.

[30] Onkendi, E., Moghaddam, MB., Oderich, GS. (2010). Internal carotid artery aneurysm in a patient with Neurofibromatosis type 1. *Vascular and Endovascular Surgery* 44, 511-514.

[31] Pearce, J. (1967). The central nervous system pathology in multiple neurofibromatosis. *Neurology* 17, 691-697.

[32] Pentecost, M., Stanley, P., Takahashi, M., Isaacs, H Jr. (1981). Aneurysms of the aorta and subclavian and vertebral arteries in neurofibromatosis. *Am J Dis Child* 135, 475-477.

[33] Peyre, M., Ozanne, A., Bhangoo, R., Pereira, V., Tadié, M., Lasjaunias, P., Parker, F. (2007). Pseudotumoral presentation of a cervical extracranial vertebral artery aneurysm in neurofibromatosis type 1: case report. *Neurosurgery* 61, E658.

[34] Riccardi, VM. (2000). The vasculopathy of NF1 and histogenesis control genes. *Clin Genet* 58, 345-347.

[35] Rasmussen, SA., Yang, Q., Friedman, JM. (2001). Mortality in Neurofibromatosis 1: an analysis using U.S. death certificates. *Am J Hum Genet* 68, 1110-1118.

[36] Shibuya, S., Tanaka, K., Saito, N., Nakajima, M., Oogi, M., Sato, K., Fukase, M. (1994). A case report of spontaneous rupture of carotid artery post caesarian section. *Journal of Tsuruoka municipal shyonai hospital* 5, 90-96.

[37] Sakamoto, S., Sumida, M., Takeshita, S., Shibukawa, M., Kiura, Y., Okazaki, T., Kurisu, K. (2009) Ruptured subclavian artery pseudo-aneurysm associated with Neurofibromatosis type 1. *Acta Neurochir* 151, 1163-1166.

[38] Schievink, WI., Piepgras, DG. (1991). Cervical vertebral artery aneurysms and arteriovenous fistulae in neurofibromatosis type 1: case reports. *Neurosurgery* 29, 760-765.

[39] Schievink, WI., Riedinger, M., Maya, MM. (2005). Frequency of incidental intracranial aneurysms in neurofibromatosis type 1. *Am J Med Genet A* 134, 45-48.

[40] Schubiger, O., Yasargil, MG. (1978). Extracranial vertebral aneurysm with neurofibromatosis. *Neuroradiology* 15, 171-173.

[41] Smith, BL., Munschauer, CE., Diamond, N., Rivera, F. (2000). Ruptured internal carotid aneurysm resulting from Neurofibromatosis: treatment with intraluminal stent graft. *J Vasc Surg* 32, 824-828.

[42] Sobota, E., Ohkuma, H., Suzuki, S. (1988). Cerebrovascular disorders associated with von Recklinghausen's Neurofibromatosis: a case report. *Neurosurgery* 22, 544-549.

[43] Takeda, H., Doi, T., Kato, H., Nagaya, S., Shirai, K., Toyoda, I., Ogura, S. (2010). A case of von Recklinghausen's disease with airway obstruction due to rupture of cervical pseudo aneurysm. *Journal of Japanese Association for Acute Medicine* 21, 84-90.

[44] Takeda, T., Takemasa, K., Takeda, A., Ohsuga, K., Shimada, K. (2002). Spontaneous arterial rupture in neurofibromatosis type 1 (NF 1); report of two cases. *Japanese Journal of Clinical Radiology* 47, 810-815.

[45] Ueda, M., Sato, H., Inoue, Y., Okawara, S., Takeda, S. Neurofibromatosis associated with distal anterior cerebral aneurysm and extracranial vertebral aneurysm. *Jpn J Stroke* 12, 301-306.47.

[46] Ushikoshi, S., Goto, K., Uda, K., Ogata, N., Takeno, Y. (1999). Vertebral arteriovenous fistula that developed in the same place as a previous ruptured aneurysm: a case report. *Surg Neurol* 51, 168-173.

[47] Viskochil, D. (2002). Genetics of Neurofibromatosis 1 and the NF1 gene. *J Child Neurol* 17, 562-570.

[48] You, MW., Kim, EJ., Choi, WS. (2011). Intracranial and extracranial fusiform aneurysms in a patient with Neurofibromatosis type 1: a case report. *Neurointervention* 6, 34-37.

In: Neurofibromatosis
Editor: Walter Romaine

ISBN: 978-1-63463-229-4
© 2015 Nova Science Publishers, Inc.

Chapter 2

HEMATOPOIETIC LINEAGES COOPERATE WITH OSTEOBLASTS IN THE INITIATION AND PROGRESSION OF NEUROFIBROMATOSIS TYPE 1 ASSOCIATED SKELETAL DEFICITS

Steven David Rhodes and Feng-Chun Yang
Herman B. Wells Center for Pediatric Research, Indiana University School
of Medicine, Indianapolis, IN, US

ABSTRACT

Neurofibromatosis type 1 (NF1), also known as von Recklinghausen disease, is a common autosomal dominant genetic disorder affecting approximately 1 in 3000 individuals worldwide. NF1 results from heritable or spontaneous mutations of the NF1 tumor suppressor gene, encoding the protein neurofibromin, which functions to negatively regulate Ras-activity. Although neurofibromas are considered the hallmark feature of NF1, up to 70 percent of NF1 patients develop both generalized and focal osseous defects including short stature, kyphoscoliosis, osteopenia/osteoporosis, fractures, and pseudarthrosis (fracture non-union). While defective osteoblast bone anabolism has been implicated as a central factor in the pathogenesis of NF1 associated skeletal deficits, recent data suggests that NF1 (Nf1) haploinsufficiency within the hematopoietic compartment, particularly in osteoclasts and myeloid progenitors, plays a pivotal role in engendering NF1 osseous manifestations. In this chapter, we review the latest data from clinical studies and murine models demonstrating a requirement for hematopoietic derived NF1 (Nf1) haploinsufficient osteoclasts and their progenitors in the pathogenesis of multiple NF1 skeletal deficits.

I. INTRODUCTION

Neurofibromatosis Type 1 (NF1)

Neurofibromatosis type 1 (NF1), first described by Friedrich von Recklinghausen in 1882, is a common autosomal dominant genetic disorder with an incidence of approximately 1 in 3,500 individuals worldwide [1]. NF1 results from heritable or spontaneous mutations of the *NF1* tumor suppressor gene. Located on the long arm of chromosome 17 [2, 3], *NF1* encodes the protein neurofibromin, which functions as a Ras GTPase activation protein (Ras-GAP), promoting the hydrolysis of active GTP-bound Ras to its inactive GDP-bound form [2, 4]. Loss of one or both functional copies of the *NF1* allele results in Ras hyperactivation in response to extracellular stimuli giving rise to the genetic disorder NF1.

In addition to the pathognomonic cutaneous and plexiform neurofibromas, extensive epidemiological study [5-7] now indicates that NF1 patients exhibit a range of malignant and non-malignant disease manifestations including café au lait macules, axillary or inguinal freckling, optic gliomas [8, 9], Lisch nodules [10], cognitive impairment [11], and cardiovascular disease [12-17]. Children with NF1 also have a 500-fold increased risk of developing juvenile myelomonocytic leukemia (JMML) due to loss of heterozygosity (LOH) of the normal *NF1* allele [18-20].

Skeletal Deficits in NF1

In addition to the aforementioned features, NF1 patients develop a range of characteristic skeletal manifestations including osteoporosis [21-26], kyphoscoliosis [27-29], short stature [30-32], macrocephaly [31], chest wall deformities [33], sphenoid wing dysplasia [6], and pseudarthrosis of the tibia [34-38]. The osseous defects can be further subclassified as either generalized or focal in nature. Generalized deficits, which include osteopenia/osteoporosis and short stature, affect greater than 50 percent of the NF1 patient population. Focal deficits, such as dystrophic scoliosis, sphenoid wing dysplasia, and tibial pseudarthrosis, occur at a lower frequency, yet are associated with significant morbidity. Collectively, the cumulative incidence of osseous defects is estimated at upwards of 70 percent of the NF1 patient population.

Osteopenia/Osteoporosis

Osteoporosis has been traditionally considered a disease of aging and was previously unrecognized as a significant complication among children and adolescents with NF1. In 2001, Illes and colleagues made a seminal observation of bone quality deficits in NF1 patients undergoing surgical correction of scoliosis, noting "very soft vertebral bone" upon intraoperative assessment [29]. These qualitative findings were corroborated by measurement of lumbar spine BMD using peripheral dual energy x-ray absorptiometry (pDEXA), revealing a mean z-score of -2.5. Moreover, the authors noted that patients with the most pronounced reductions in BMD tended to have increased severity of scoliosis [29], a finding which was subsequently validated in a larger cross-sectional study of 104 NF1 patients [21]. Serum deoxypyridinoline (Dpd)/pyridinoline (Pyd) ratios are an established biomarker of bone resorption that is often increased in high bone turnover states including osteoporosis, Paget's disease, and hyperparathyroidism [39-41]. Consistent with these findings, children and adolescents with NF1 also exhibit significantly increased Dpd/Pyd ratios [42]. A consensus of published literature indicates that upwards of 50 percent of children and adolescents with NF1 suffer from osteopenia/osteoporosis as defined by clinical criteria [21, 23-25].

Until recently, the sequelae of osteopenia/osteoporosis in the NF1 patient population had remained unknown. It has been hypothesized that increased bone resorption and reduced BMD could lead to the accumulation of clinically undetected microfractures in patients with NF1, compromising the mechanical integrity of bone later in life. In 2009, Tucker and colleagues reported that the incidence of fracture among adults with NF1 was markedly increased as compared to unaffected siblings and spouses [26]. 41 fractures were documented among 24 out of 72 NF1 patients, as compared to just six fractures among six individuals out of 73 unaffected siblings. Moreover, among the NF1 patient cohort, 24 pathological fractures (associated with minimal trauma) were documented in 14 individuals, whereas no pathological fractures were reported in the unaffected cohort [26]. More recently, a controlled study of 460 neurofibromatosis patients conducted in Finland [43] confirmed that adults with NF1 ages 41 years and older had a 5.2-fold increased risk of fracture versus age-matched controls without NF1. Strikingly, even children with NF1 ages 17 and under had a 3.4-fold increased risk ratio for fractures [43], reinforcing that the osteoporotic manifestations of NF1 warrant early clinical intervention.

Spinal Deformities

Gould and Weiss first commented on the increased incidence of spinal deformities among NF1 patients in the early 1900s [44, 45]. Varying clinical reports suggest that between 10 and 77 percent of the NF1 patient population exhibit kyphoscoliosis [46-48]. Moreover, approximately 2% of all pediatric scoliosis cases are associated with NF1 [49]. Scoliosis can be further defined as either dystrophic or non-dystrophic based on the presence or absence of characteristic radiographic features [50]. Non-dystrophic scoliosis in NF1 is radiographically indistinguishable from idiopathic scoliosis but presents earlier and is associated with an increased incidence of pseudarthrosis following spinal fusion [51]. Dystrophic scoliosis is characterized by dysplastic osseous anomalies with rapid onset and progression. The hallmark radiographic features associated with dystrophic scoliosis in NF1 include rib penciling, short-segment sharply angulated curves involving four to six vertebrae, vertebral rotation, scalloping of the vertebral margins, spindling of the transverse processes, pedicle defects, and widening of the spinal canal [50, 52]. Dystrophic scoliosis is associated with significant morbidity in children and adolescents with NF1 due to the potential for rapid degeneration to neurological impairment. Orthopedic manipulation is also associated with an increased risk of pseudarthrosis in the affected vertebrae following surgical intervention [27, 53].

Pseudarthrosis

Congenital pseudarthrosis, first documented by James Paget in 1891, is a rare orthopedic condition characterized by anterolateral tibial bowing with tapering at the defective site [54]. Although the cumulative incidence of congenital pseudarthrosis is only 1:140,000-1:250,000 individuals among the general population [55], remarkably, it is estimated that 50-80% of all congenital tibial pseudarthrosis cases involve mutations in *NF1* [56-59].

Fractures may occur spontaneously or following minimal trauma. Bone healing is insufficient, resulting in persistent fibrous non-union even after multiple surgeries. Elective limb amputation is often required for the affected child to regain mobility due to limited and currently ineffective therapies.

Tissues surgically excised from NF1 pseudarthrosis lesions exhibit a mesenchymal lineage phenotype, expressing the cell surface markers CD44 and CD105, but are negative for CD45 and CD14 [60]. They express BMP receptors, although fail to undergo osteoblastic differentiation in response to exogenous BMP [60]. Osteoclast infiltration is another prominent histological feature [59, 61, 62]. Cho and colleagues demonstrated that mesenchymal cells cultured *ex vivo* from pseudarthrosis tissue expressed supraphysiologic levels of receptor activator of nuclear factor kappa-B ligand (RANKL) while secreting lower levels of osteoprotegerin (OPG) as compared to control tibial periosteal cells, thereby potentiating osteoclast differentiation of Raw264.7 cells in co-culture experiments [60].

Brief Chapter Overview

Although investigation of the cellular and molecular etiology of NF1 skeletal deficits remains in its infancy, clinical and animal model studies imply that the genesis of NF1 associated skeletal anomalies involves heterotypic interaction of multiple cell lineages with varying *NF1* gene dose. Here we review the evidence demonstrating that *NF1*(*Nf1*) haploinsufficient bone marrow derived myeloid progenitors and osteoclasts cooperate with *Nf1* deficient mesenchymal stem cells (MSCs)/osteoblasts to engender multiple NF1 osseous deficits including osteoporosis and tibial fracture non-union (pseudarthrosis).

II. Skeletal Homeostasis and Hematopoiesis Are Interdependent

The interplay between bone and the hematopoietic system has been a focal point of intensive investigation during recent years. Discovery of reciprocal interactions between mesenchymal stem cells (MSCs)/osteoblasts and hematopoietic stem cells (HSCs) within a restricted microenvironment termed the niche [63-69] has heightened our awareness of the interdependence of skeletal homeostasis and hematopoiesis. Indeed, the bone and blood do not exist in isolation; rather, these tissues are bidirectionally interrelated, such that pathologies arising in one system can adversely affect the other and vice versa.

Hematopoietic Derived Myeloid Cells/Osteoclasts Are the Primary Mediators of Bone Resorption

Hematopoietic stem cells (HSCs) are self-renewing, multipotential cells which give rise to all constituents of the hematopoietic system including erythrocytes, megakaryocytes, myeloid cells, and lymphocytes. Beyond HSCs, a restriction of cell fates occurs at the multipotent progenitor stage, where cells are delineated as either common myeloid or lymphoid progenitors, which give rise to both B- and T-lymphocytes. Common myeloid progenitor cells (CMPs) can further differentiate to either granulocyte macrophage progenitors (GMPs), which give rise to mast cells, eosinophils, neutrophils, monocyte /macrophages, or megakaryocyte/erythroid progenitors, which ultimately give rise to platelets and red blood cells [70]. Aside from their canonical roles in blood and the immune system, the interaction of these hematopoietic constituents with bone is now recognized to have a profound impact on skeletal health and disease.

Osteoclasts are specialized monocyte/macrophages that arise from HSCs and are the primary cell type responsible for bone resorption. The capacity of osteoclast progenitors to proliferate, differentiate, adhere, and resorb the bone matrix is critical to the maintenance of skeletal homeostasis. Disorders of low bone mass, such as osteoporosis, are typically associated with enhanced osteoclast recruitment and bone erosive activity. By contrast, arrest of osteoclastogenesis or disruption of resorptive function can lead to pathological increases in bone mass, termed osteopetrosis.

Differentiation of myelomoncytic progenitor cells to mature, bone resorptive osteoclasts is regulated by mechanisms both intrinsic and extrinsic to the cell. The cytokines macrophage-colony stimulating factor (M-CSF) [71] and receptor activator of nuclear factor κB ligand (RANK-L) [72, 73] are indispensable for macrophage and osteoclast development. Receptor binding of M-CSF and RANK-L leads to activation of both MAPK and PI3K signaling pathways which potentiate osteoclast differentiation, survival, and cytoskeletal reorganization [74]. Within the osteoclast, RANK recruitment of the adaptor protein TNF receptor-associated factor 6 (TRAF6) is critical for the NF κB dependent activation of osteoclast specific genes [75].

Mice lacking M-CSF (o*p/op*) exhibit severe osteopetrosis due to an absence of both osteoclasts and macrophages [76]. Moreover adoptive transfer of wild-type (WT) hematopoietic cells to osteopetrotic *op/op* recipient mice is insufficient to correct the phenotype, implying that the failure of macrophage/osteoclast differentiation in the *op/op* mouse is contingent on the extrinsic absence of M-CSF, as opposed to an intrinsic cellular defect [76]. Likewise, genetic ablation of RANK-L [77] or the *Tnfrsf11a* gene encoding RANK leads to a similar phenotype [72, 78] due to the inability of monocyte/macrophages to undergo terminal osteoclast differentiation. As osteoblasts continue to mineralize new matrix in the absence of bone resorption, they fill up the niche, eliminating the space required to maintain hematopoiesis. Anemia, thrombocytopenia, and a compromised immune response to infection are common late stage symptoms of malignant osteopetrosis. In 1980, Coccia and colleagues reported the first successful cure of this otherwise fatal disorder by bone marrow transplantation, restoring osteoclast resorptive activity and hematopoiesis [79].

By contrast, mice lacking osteoprotegerin (OPG), a soluble 'decoy receptor' for RANK-L, exhibit profound osteoporosis due to increased osteolytic activity [80]. Aside from mutations in the M-CSF and RANK-L receptor/ligand, alterations in the intracellular response of myelomonocytic precursors to M-CSF and RANKL signals is an important intracellular mechanism by which deregulated osteoclast recruitment and function can occur. As an illustration of this concept, the Src homology (SH) 2-containing inositol-5-phosphatase (SHIP) protein attenuates PI3K signaling by dephosphorylating its major substrate, phosphatidylinositol 3,4,5-triphosphate (PIP3) [81, 82]. *SHIP* deficient mice exhibit increased osteoclast differentiation, severe osteoporosis, and acquire myeloproliferative disease due to hypersensitivity to multiple hematopoietic growth factors mediated by uncontrolled PI3K signaling [83]. Evidence now suggests that neurofibromin's regulation of p21-Ras activity in HSCs and myeloid progenitor cells is another pivotal axis regulating osteoclast recruitment/function and this concept will be discussed at length in subsequent sections of this chapter.

Beyond macrophages and osteoclasts, mast cells are another myeloid lineage derived from the granulocyte monocyte progenitor (GMP) which have been recognized to regulate bone homeostasis, albeit indirectly. The concept that mast cells and their secreted products may modulate bone turnover is supported by a number of studies. Comparing *W/W* mast cell deficient mice to wild-type (WT) controls, Silberstein and colleagues demonstrated that mice lacking mast cells exhibited a decreased rate of osteoclastic bone resorption as well as diminished synthesis of new bone matrix by osteoblasts [84]. Histamine, a major mast cell mediator released during degranulation, has also been shown to play an important role in osteoclast resorptive activity. Mice with targeted disruption of histamine decarboxylase, the enzyme responsible for histamine production, exhibit increased bone mass and reduced osteoclast numbers [85]. Analogously, pharmacologic blockade of histamine receptors has been shown to inhibit osteoclastogenesis and restorptive activity, thereby preventing bone loss in ovariectomized rats [86, 87]. Clinically, patients with systemic mastocytosis exhibit generalized osteopenia, with evidence of increased osteoclast infiltration localized to focal areas of mast cell accumulation within the bone marrow [88, 89]. While *Nf1* haploinsufficient (*Nf1$^{+/-}$*) mast cells have been demonstrated to exhibit multiple gain-in-functions [90], their potential contribution to osteopenia and other skeletal deficits in NF1 remains unclear. A number of other hematopoietic lineages including B-cells [91], T-cells [92], and megakaryocytes [93, 94] have also been shown to affect bone remodeling; however, a detailed discussion of the role of these lineages in the maintenance of bone homeostasis is beyond the scope of this discussion.

Osteoblast – Osteoclast Cross Talk in Bone Homeostasis

The concept that osteoblasts may regulate osteoclast bone resorptive activity through hormonal cross-talk was first proposed by Rodan and Martin in 1981 [95]. In fact, prior to elucidation of RANK-L in the late 1990s [72, 73], the generation of osteoclasts from bone marrow mononuclear cells *in vitro* was primarily accomplished through osteoblast/stromal cell co-culture methods. Osteoblasts are now recognized as the primary source of multiple osteoclastogenic cytokines including M-CSF [96], RANK-L [72, 73], and osteoprotegerin (OPG) [97]. Additionally, osteoblasts have been shown to secrete a number of chemotactic cytokines stimulating the recruitment of monocytes and osteoclast progenitors to the bone surface including monocyte chemotactic protein 1 (MCP1) [98] and osteopontin (OPN) [99]. In NF1, hypersecretion of OPN by *Nf1* mutant osteoblasts [100] together with alterations in the RANK-L/OPG cytokine ratio [101] have been hypothesized to contribute significantly to enhancing osteoclast recruitment and bone catabolic activity *in vivo*.

The constitutive processes of osteoclast bone resorption and formation of new bone matrix by osteoblasts are linked in space and time by osteoblast secreted factors, which are stored in the bone matrix, and subsequently liberated by osteoclasts during bone resorption. The critical role of transforming growth factor-beta1 (TGF-β1) as a master regulator of the spatiotemporal coupling of bone remodeling was recently demonstrated in a mouse model recapitulating multiple osseous features of Camurati-Engelmann Disease (CED) associated with increased levels of active TGF-β1 in the bone matrix [102]. Intriguingly, there is considerable phenotypic overlap between the characteristic skeletal manifestations of NF1 with those found in other TGF-β associated disorders including Loeys-Dietz syndrome [103-106], Marfan syndrome [107-111], and CED [112]. Indeed, recent studies have confirmed that hyperactive transforming growth factor-β1 signaling indeed plays a critical role in the pathogenesis of multiple NF1 associated osseous deficits including osteoporosis and tibial fracture non-union (pseudarthrosis) [113], and will be discussed subsequently in this chapter.

Emerging evidence now demonstrates that osteoblast – osteoclast cross-talk is not merely unidirectional. In a reciprocal fashion, osteoclasts also possess the capacity to influence osteoblast bone formation. The existence of such bidirectional signaling interactions was first reported in 2006 by Zhao and colleagues, whereby forward signaling through EphB4 into osteoblast precursors enhances osteoblast differentiation while reverse signaling through ephrinB2 suppresses osteoclast differentiation [114]. Most recently, Negishi-Koga et al. demonstrated that binding of osteoclast expressed semaphorin 4D (Sema4D) to the Plexin-B1 receptor on osteoblasts inhibits bone formation, thereby decoupling the remodeling process [115]. The role of bidirectional osteoblast-osteoclast communication through ephrins, semaphorins or other novel cross-talk mechanisms in the pathogenesis of NF1 skeletal defects have yet to be elucidated.

III. *NF1* GENE DOSE PIVOTALLY REGULATES MYELOID CELL FATE AND FUNCTION

Myeloid cell anomalies occur frequently in NF1 patients. Children with NF1 have a 500-fold increased incidence of juvenile myelomonocytic leukemia (JMML) due to loss of *NF1* heterozygosity (LOH) in the bone marrow [18-20]. Consistent with these findings, transplantation of hematopoietic cells from the fetal livers of *Nf1*$^{-/-}$ mice results uniformly in the development of myeloproliferative disease (MPD) which is closely reminiscent of JMML [116-119]. Chimerisim analyses from competitive repopulation assays performed by Zhang et al. further delineate that the growth advantage conferred by *Nf1* inactivation varies in a cell-type specific fashion, resulting in myeloid lineage skewing within the hematopoietic compartment [118]. On a mechanistic level, human JMML cells and *Nf1*$^{-/-}$ myeloid progenitors demonstrate a markedly increased proliferative response to multiple cytokines [120] including granulocyte macrophage-colony stimulating factor (GM-CSF), interleukin-3 (IL-3), and stem cell factor (SCF), which promote leukemogenesis via hyperactive Ras-Raf-Mek-Erk signaling [121, 122]. Still, the potential effects of *Nf1* LOH within the hematopoietic compartment on skeletal development and homeostasis remain to be determined.

IV. *NF1* HAPLOINSUFFICIENT HEMATOPOIETIC CELLS COOPERATE TO ENGENDER MULTIPLE NF1 SKELETAL ANOMALIES IN MICE

Nf1 gene dose is critical to regulating myeloid cell fate and function. Haploinsufficient or nullizygous loss of *Nf1* in myeloid cells can engender characteristic NF1 associated phenotypes including plexiform neurfibromas [123], neointima formation [124, 125], and myeloproliferative disease (JMML) as reviewed above. The remainder of this chapter will discuss emerging evidence indicating that cooperative interactions between *Nf1* deficient mesenchymal cells/osteoblasts and *Nf1* haploinsufficient hematopoietic cells are required to perpetuate NF1 osseous manifestations in mice by enhancing osteoclastogenesis and osteolytic activity. These findings have important implications for the development of novel therapeutic strategies to treat NF1 associated skeletal anomalies including osteoporosis and tibial pseudarthrosis which have been historically refractory to conventional anti-resorptive therapies.

Modeling NF1 Skeletal Dysplasia in the Mouse

Mouse models have been critical for gleaning insight into the role of *Nf1* in bone biology and as a platform for preclinical testing of potential pharmacologic therapies. *Nf1*$^{-/-}$ mice are not suitable for bone studies as they die *in utero* prior to embryonic day 13 due to cardiac developmental abnormalities [126]. Additionally, adoptive transfer of hematopoietic cells from $Nf1^{-/-}$ fetal livers has been shown to consistently induce myeloproliferative disease (MPD) reminiscent of JMML as discussed previously [116, 120].

$Nf1^{+/-}$ mice are viable into adulthood and have been utilized extensively in the study of NF1 associated bone defects. Bone marrow mononuclear cells cultured *ex vivo* from $Nf1^{+/-}$ mice and human NF1 patients exhibit increased propensity for osteoclast differentiation and display multiple osteoclast gain-in-functions including increased proliferation, survival, and bone resorption [127-129] which are associated with elevated p21Ras-GTP and Akt phosphorylation in response to M-CSF and RANK-L stimulation. Genetic intercross with mice deficient in class 1a PI3K (p85α) is sufficient to attenuate Akt phosphorylation and normalize aberrant $Nf1^{+/-}$ osteoclast functions [127]. Collectively, these data indicate that hyperactivity of p21-Ras and PI3K cooperate to alter *Nf1* haploinsufficient osteoclast functions.

Rho GTPases act as key molecular gatekeepers downstream of hyperactivated Ras and PI3K, cycling between inactive-GDP and active-GTP-bound forms to modulate osteoclast cytoskeletal functions. Yan and colleagues demonstrated that the Rho-GTPase Rac1 is a critical Ras effector mediating aberrant osteoclast migration and f-actin rearrangement within $Nf1^{+/-}$ osteoclast podosomes [130]. Genetic disruption of *Rac1* in $Nf1^{+/-}$ mice attenuated extracellular signal-regulated kinase 1/2 (Erk1/2) phosphorylation while normalizing the cytoskeletal dynamics and bone resorptive activity of *Nf1* haploinsufficient osteoclasts. Application of a pharmacologic MEK inhibitor (PD98059) yielded analogous results, indicating a pivotal role for cross-talk between PI3K-Rac1 signaling and the Ras-Raf-MEK-Erk axis in perpetuating $Nf1^{+/-}$ osteoclast gain-in functions [130].

The significance of increased Erk1/2 biochemical activity in *Nf1* haploinsufficient osteoclasts is corroborated by recent functional studies regarding the differential and reciprocal roles of Erk1/2 isoforms in osteoclast biology [131, 132]. He et al. demonstrated that Erk1 as compared to Erk2, plays a preponderant role as a positive regulator of osteoclast formation and bone resorptive functions. $Erk1^{-/-}$ mice exhibit reduced osteoclast progenitor numbers, diminished resorptive capacity, and impaired adhesion and migration in response to M-CSF stimulation [131]. The marrow autonomous nature of *Erk1* dependent osteoclast functions was further validated by reconstituting the hematopoietic system of WT mice with *Erk1* deficient bone marrow. Consistent with the phenotype of $Erk1^{-/-}$ mice, WT hosts transplanted with

$Erk1^{-/-}$ bone marrow mononuclear cells (BMMNCs) demonstrated increased bone mass as compared to controls reconstituted with either WT or $Erk2^{-/-}$ BMMNCs [131].

Studies utilizing the $Nf1^{+/-}$ mouse model have also demonstrated that neurofibromin plays a critical role in the capacity of mesenchymal stem cells (MSCs) to undergo osteoblast differentiation. While $Nf1^{+/-}$ MSCs exhibit increased proliferation and colony forming unit-fibroblast (CFU-F), their propensity to undergo osteoblast differentiation in response to osteogenic stimuli is significantly impaired [133]. Retroviral transduction of $Nf1^{+/-}$ MSPCs with the human full-length $NF1$ GTPase activating related domain ($NF1$ GRD) for p21-Ras was sufficient to rescue osteoblast differentiation, demonstrating the Ras-dependent nature of these cellular defects [133].

Although osteoclasts and osteoblasts cultured *ex vivo* from $Nf1^{+/-}$ mice exhibit aberrant differentiation and function, these animals do not spontaneously develop any of the pathognomonic skeletal manifestations of NF1 such as osteoporosis, scoliosis, or pseudarthrosis observed in the human disease [134]. Nonetheless, Yang and colleagues demonstrated that the consequences of $Nf1$ haploinsufficiency can be unmasked *in vivo* following ovariectomy (OVX) induced pro-resorptive challenge, whereby $Nf1^{+/-}$ mice lose bone mass at nearly double the rate of WT controls [127]. These *in vivo* data provided the first evidence regarding the putative role of $Nf1$ haploinsufficiency in perpetuating osteoclast gain-in functions in an animal model of NF1 associated osteoporosis. Subsequently, Schindeler et al. reported the healing of distal tibial fractures to be significantly impaired in $Nf1^{+/-}$ mice, exhibiting many of the hallmark pathological features of tibial pseudarthrosis in human NF1 including delayed cartilage removal, invasion of fibrous tissue, deficient bone anabolism, and excessive osteoclast bone catabolic activity [135]. However, the lack of a prominent bone phenotype in these animals in the absence of such stressors suggests that $Nf1$ heterozygosity alone is insufficient to spontaneously recapitulate the full spectrum of osseous manifestations observed in the human disease.

In an effort to more accurately phenocopy the spectrum of NF1 osseous deficits in a murine model, various laboratories have utilized Cre/loxP technology to achieve conditional $Nf1$ nullizygosity in select lineages within the mesenchymal hierarchy. This approach was initially adopted by Elefteriou and colleagues to achieve biallelic inactivation of $Nf1$ in osteoblasts by intercrossing $Nf1^{flox/flox}$ mice with α1(I) Collagen Cre (*Col2.3Cre*) transgenic mice. Paradoxically, however, the authors found that these mice exhibited increased bone mass in the vertebral spine [101] – a phenotype which is the antithesis of the osteoporotic features seen in the human disease. Intriguingly, the same mice have also been reported to exhibit recalcitrant bone healing in a tibial fracture repair model due to deficient osteoblast differentiation [136]. Although the reasons for these discrepancies remain unclear, studies in the $Nf1^{flox/flox}$;Col2.3Cre murine model indicate that conditional $Nf1$ nullizygosity in mature osteoblasts is insufficient to promote the spontaneous genesis of cardinal NF1 osseous manifestations.

The failure of single lineage conditional knockout models to recapitulate the full spectrum of NF1 skeletal defects suggests that these manifestations may indeed require the heterotypic interaction of multiple cell lineages with varying gene dose. Consistent with this hypothesis, Stevenson et al. published a seminal case report documenting two patients with localized loss of $NF1$ heterozygosity (LOH) in pseudathrotic bone tissue microdissected the lesion site [137]. Further corroborating these data, a more recent case series documented localized $NF1$ LOH in four out of 16 pseudarthrosis patients [138]. Collectively, these findings indicate that localized biallelic $NF1$ inactivation in either osteoblasts or mesenchymal progenitor cells may cooperate with other $NF1$ haploinsufficient lineages in the bone microenvironment to engender recalcitrant bone repair in at least a subset of patients with pseudarthrosis.

To recapitulate this genetic framework in an animal model, Wu and colleagues generated transgenic $Nf1^{flox/-}$;PeriCre and $Nf1^{flox/-}$;Col2.3Cre mice, harboring $Nf1$ nullizygous MSCs and osteoblasts, respectively, on a $Nf1$ heterozygous background. These strains exhibited multiple skeletal phenotypes observed in NF1 patients, including osteoporosis [139], non-dystrophic and dystrophic vertebral deficits [140], and tibial fracture non-union (pseudarthrosis) [139]. Intriguingly, similar phenotypes were not observed in $Nf1^{flox/flox}$;Col2.3Cre and $Nf1^{flox/flox}$;PeriCre mice (harboring conditional nullizygous osteoblasts/MSCs on a WT background) [139], suggesting that genesis of these osseous deficits requires cooperative interactions between $Nf1$ null mesenchymal stem cells/osteoblasts and at least a subset of other $Nf1$ heterozygous cells within the bone microenvironment.

Critical Role for $Nf1$ Haploinsufficient Hematopoietic Cells in the Genesis of NF1 Osseous Deficits

To evaluate whether $Nf1$ haploinsufficiency in the hematopoietic compartment may cooperate with $Nf1$ nullizygous osteoblasts to engender bone mass deficits and tibial fracture non-union in $Nf1^{flox/-};Col2.3Cre$ mice, Wu and colleagues proceeded to transplant bone marrow mononuclear cells (BMMNCs) from either WT or $Nf1^{+/-}$ donor mice into lethally irradiated $Nf1^{flox/-};Col2.3Cre$ or $Nf1^{flox/flox};Col2.3Cre$ recipients [139]. The authors demonstrated both radiographically and histologically that fracture healing in $Nf1^{flox/flox};Col2.3Cre$ mice reconstituted with $Nf1^{+/-}$ marrow was significantly impaired relative to those receiving WT bone marrow cells. Micro-computed tomographic (μCT) analysis revealed a significant reduction in BV/TV fraction in $Nf1^{flox/flox};Col2.3Cre$ recipients transplanted with $Nf1^{+/-}$ bone marrow cells versus controls receiving WT bone marrow. Conversely, transplantation of WT bone marrow prevented tibial fracture non-union normally observed in $Nf1^{flox/-};Col2.3Cre$ mice. Collectively, these data provide rigorous evidence that $Nf1$ haploinsufficiency in at least a subset of hematopoietic lineages within the bone microenvironment is integral to the pathogenesis of bone mass deficits and tibial fracture non-union in $Nf1^{flox/-};Col2.3Cre$ mice. Still, the culprit lineage(s) within the $Nf1$ haploinsufficient hematopoietic system that are critical to the genesis of these phenotypes remain to be fully delineated.

Hematopoietic-derived osteoclasts are abundantly present in pseudarthrotic tissues of NF1 patients [59, 61, 62] and in mouse models of the disease [135, 136, 139, 141, 142]. Mononuclear cells cultured *ex vivo* from the peripheral blood of NF1 patients [127-129] and the bone marrow of $Nf1^{+/-}$ mice [127, 130] exhibit enhanced osteoclast differentiation and bone resorptive capacity, driven by Ras-mediated hypersensitivity to M-CSF and RANKL [127]. Collectively, these observations implicate $Nf1^{+/-}$ myeloid progenitor cells and/or osteoclasts as the culprit hematopoietic mediators of bone mass deficits and tibial fracture non-union in the NF1 murine model. In fact, Alanne and colleagues recently reported that transgenic mice harboring conditional $Nf1$ nullizygous ($Nf1^{-/-}$) osteoclasts driven by $TRAPCre$, exhibit increased osteolytic activity and aberrant actin ring formation *in vitro* [143]. In addition, $Nf1^{flox/flox};TRAPCre$ mice exhibit a number of extra-osseous features including splenomegaly and megakaryocytosis [143] which are reminiscent of the juvenile myelomonocytic leukemia (JMML)-like myeloproliferative disease (MPD) phenotypes which occur following $Nf1$ loss of heterozygosity (LOH) in the hematopoietic compartment [116-119]. These findings are suggestive of $TRAPCre$ mediated $Nf1$ recombination in relatively primitive myeloid osteoclast precursors as previously described [144]. While the physiological relevance of the $Nf1^{flox/flox};TRAPCre$ model is questionable given that NF1 patients suffering from osteoporosis typically retain a single functional *NF1* allele in the hematopoietic compartment, these data nonetheless provide critical insight regarding the stage of myeloid/osteoclast differentiation at which loss of *Nf1* is permissive to osteoclast hyperactivity. Further studies using Cre promoters specific to myeloid progenitors (eg. *LysMCre* [145]) to dissect the cell autonomous consequences of *Nf1* haploinsufficiency within specific hematopoietic cell lineages are warranted. In sum, these data provide insights regarding the step-wise role of *Nf1* in regulating myeloid differentiation, osteoclast gain-in-functions, and the putative contribution of these lineages to the genesis of bone mass deficits and tibial fracture non-union in transgenic animal models of the human disease.

The concept that $Nf1^{+/-}$ bone marrow cells of the myelomonocytic lineage play a pivotal role in the pathogenesis of tibial fracture non-union has been challenged by a recent pseudarthrosis model developed by El-Hoss and colleagues which utilizes the injection of a Cre-expressing adenovirus (AdCre) to locally inactivate floxed *Nf1* alleles within the fracture site [146]. When comparing the healing rate of fractures generated in $Nf1^{flox/flox}$ versus $Nf1^{flox/-}$ mice following injection of AdCre, there was no significant difference in the rate of fracture repair between the two strains. Although a robust model for recapitulating multiple histopathological features of the human disease, the ability to evaluate the consequences of *Nf1* gene dose within the bone microenvironment is limited by this approach due to the inherent lack of selectivity associated with AdCre injection, whereby Cre-mediated recombination of the floxed *Nf1* allele(s) will occur non-specifically in all cell types present within the lesion including bone marrow, stroma, vasculature, etc. In effect, AdCre injection renders $Nf1^{flox/flox}$ and $Nf1^{flox/-}$ strains genetically equivalent within the local fracture site, whereby all cells transduced with AdCre effectively become *Nf1* nullizygous – thus explaining why equivocal results were likely obtained when comparing the $Nf1^{flox/flox}$ and $Nf1^{flox/-}$ strains following AdCre injection.

Of note, widespread biallelic recombination of *Nf1* in either undifferentiated limb bud mesenchyme driven by *Prx1Cre* [141] or osteochondroprogneitor cells driven by *Col2a1Cre* (collagen, type II, alpha 1 promotor) [142] results in a broad spectrum of osseous anomalies. $Nf1^{flox/flox};Prx1Cre$ mice exhibit severe runting, fusion of the hip joints, malformed limbs, and tibial bowing associated with increased cortical bone porosity and failure of both osteoblast and chondrocyte differentiation [141]. In addition to these phenotypes, $Nf1^{flox/flox};Col2a1Cre$ mice exhibit bone mass deficits, profound kyphoscoliosis, and defects in intervertebral disc (IVD) formation at nearly every level of the vertebral column [142]. Thus, early and widespread loss of *Nf1* function in limb bud mesenchyme or osteochondroprogenitor cells circumvents the requirement for cooperative interactions between *Nf1* nullizygous osteoblasts and $Nf1^{+/-}$ hematopoietic cells in the genesis of bone mass deficits and tibial fracture non-union in the $Nf1^{flox/-};Col2.3Cre$ mouse model. However, the presence of widespread IVD defects, joint anomalies, and severe short stature which are not characteristic features of the human disease, together with the exceedingly high penetrance of osseous phenotypes observed in the $Nf1^{flox/flox};Prx1Cre$ and $Nf1^{flox/flox};Col2a1Cre$ models raises questions as to the physiological relevance of diffuse biallelic *Nf1* inactivation at such a primitive developmental stage. While skeletal anomalies in human NF1 patients occur in the context of a systemic $NF1^{+/-}$ genetic background, the putative microenvironment effect of $Nf1^{+/-}$ bone marrow and stromal cells remains to be examined in the $Nf1^{flox/flox};Prx1Cre$ and $Nf1^{flox/flox};Col2a1Cre$ models. Regardless of the aforementioned limitations, these models nonetheless provide fundamental insights regarding the potential cell of origin for *NF1* loss of heterozygosity (LOH) within the mesenchymal compartment in the genesis of NF1 skeletal anomalies.

V. THERAPEUTIC IMPLICATIONS IN THE TREATMENT OF NF1 SKELETAL DISEASE

Evidence that cooperative interactions between *Nf1* deficient mesenchymal cells/osteoblasts and hematopoietic derived *Nf1* myeloid progenitor cells are pivotal to engendering NF1 osseous deficits has important therapeutic implications for the treatment of osteoporosis, tibial pseudarthrosis, and other NF1 skeletal anomalies which have been historically refractory to conventional anti-resorptive therapies. Bisphosphonates have been the mainstay of osteoporosis therapy for more than two decades. These agents function by accumulating in the bone matrix and inducing apoptosis of terminally differentiated osteoclasts as they resorb bone [147]. Bisphosphonates can be further subcategorized as either amino or non-amino bisphosphonates based on their molecular structure and mechanism of action. Non-amino-bisphosphates, such as clodronate, disrupt mitochondrial functions and induce osteoclast apoptosis by the generation of toxic ATP analogous. By contrast, amino-bisphosphonates including alendronate and zoledronic acid induce cell death by inhibiting the farnesyllation of small GTPases such as Ras, Rac and Rho [147].

Intriguingly, Heervä and colleagues demonstrated that osteoclasts cultured *ex vivo* from human NF1 patients display marked insensitivity to bisphosphonate mediated apoptosis [148]. Consistent with these data, a recent clinical study involving a small cohort of NF1 patients undergoing a 23-month course of bisphosphonate therapy did not show significant increases in BMD [149]. Indeed, there are currently no clinical trials which support the use of traditional anti-resorptive therapies to treat NF1 associated bone mass deficits [35]. Despite evidence of reduced Vitamin D levels in a subset of NF1 patients [150], supplementation with calcium and Vitamin D did not significantly improve BMD z-scores after 2 years follow-up [151]. As recent clinical data has confirmed that NF1 patients suffering from osteopenia/osteoporosis are at a substantially increased risk of fracture [26, 43], there is thus a significant unmet need for devising alternative strategies to augment bone mineral density in these individuals. This is particularly relevant in the case of tibial pseudarthrosis, where patients often undergo elective limb amputation to regain mobility after multiple failed surgical interventions.

Recent insights demonstrating the pivotal role of hematopoietic *Nf1* halpoinsufficient osteoclast progenitors in the pathogenesis of bone mass deficits and fracture non-union in NF1 mouse models suggest that therapies targeting osteoclast precursor cells at a more primitive differentiative stage may hold unique therapeutic promise for treating osteoporosis and other NF1 skeletal maladies resulting from excess osteolytic activity. He et al. demonstrated that $Nf1^{+/-}$ osteoclast progenitors exhibit marked hypersensitivity to M-CSF binding to the c-Fms receptor, promoting multiple osteoclast gain-in-functions including migration, adhesion, and bone resorptive capacity which were associated with hyperactivation of the downstream effectors Erk1/2 and p90rsk [152]. Administration of PLX3397, a pharmacologic inhibitor of c-Fms receptor tyrosine kinase activity, was sufficient to mitigate $Nf1^{+/-}$ osteoclast hyperactivity *in vitro*, while preventing accelerated bone loss in $Nf1^{+/-}$ mice following ovariectomy induced pro-resorptive stress [152].

Given that cooperative interactions among local *Nf1*-nullizygous osteoprogenitors and *Nf1* haploinsufficient osteoclasts of the bone marrow play a key role in perpetuating deregulated bone turnover in NF1, therapies aimed at restoring the functional balance between osteoclast bone resorption and osteoblast bone anabolic activity may hold advantages over traditional monotherapies targeting either the osteoclast or osteoblast alone. There is now preclinical and clinical data to suggest that combination therapy with rhBMP-2 plus a bisphosphonate can enhance the rate of tibial fracture healing both in $Nf1^{+/-}$ mice as well human NF1 pseudarthrosis patients [153, 154]. Nonetheless, pathway specific, targeted agents directed at augmenting osteoblast bone formation and curtailing osteoclast catabolic activity remain the ultimate goal of therapy. The utility of lovastatin as an inhibitor of Ras prenylation required for membrane targeting has been explored in a number of NF1 pseudarthrosis animal models with positive results [136, 142, 155]. Given that *NF1* gene inactivation leads to hyperactivation of the Ras-MEK-MAPK signaling pathway, it has been hypothesized that pharmacologic MEK inhibition may prove beneficial in augmenting bone healing and quality. Indeed, administration of the pharmacologic MEK inhibitor PD98059 significantly improved the rate of tibial fracture healing in $Nf1^{flox/-}$;*Col2.3Cre* mice [156]. This phenotype was associated with enhanced osteoblast differentiation and diminished osteoclastogensis in response to PD98059 treatment. El-Hoss and colleagues subsequently reported that the combination of rhBMP and the MEK inhibitor PD0325901 could augment fracture bone volume but did not substantially reduce fibrosis in a tibial psuedarthrosis model featuring localized biallelic *Nf1* inactivation driven by AdCre injection into a closed tibial fracture [157].

Intrigued by the considerable phenotypic overlap between the characteristic skeletal manifestations of NF1 with those found in other TGF-β associated disorders including Loeys-Dietz syndrome [103-106], Marfan syndrome [107-111], and Camurati-Engelmann disease [112], Rhodes and colleagues proceeded to test whether targeting TGF-β as a master regulator in the spatiotemporal coupling of bone remodeling may hold therapeutic value in the treatment of NF1 associated osseous manifestations [113]. The authors delineated a mechanism by which p21-Ras dependent hyperactivation of the canonical TGF-β1-Smad pathway potentiates *Nf1* haploinsufficient osteoclast gain-in-functions while suppressing bone anabolic activity of *Nf1* deficient osteoblasts, thereby decoupling bone resorption from formation. In accordance with these findings, pharmacologic TβRI kinase inhibition was sufficient to rescue bone mass deficits and prevent tibial fracture non-union in a transgenic mouse model recapitulating multiple osseous features of the human disease [113].

Consistent with these data, TGF-β is known to stimulate ERK activation in chondrocytes, leading to accumulation of pyrophosphate PPi, a potent inhibitor of bone mineralization. Intriguingly, de la Croix Ndong and colleagues recently demonstrated that *Nf1* deletion in osteochondroprogenitor cells leads to supraphysiologic accumulation of PPi in bone forming cells.

Asfotase-α enzyme therapy, aimed at reducing PPi concentrations rescued short stature and augmented bone mineralization and strength in mice harboring *Nf1* deficient osteochondroprogenitors [158]. Clinical pilot studies and early phase trials are needed to begin evaluating the efficacy of these and other novel therapeutic approaches in the treatment of NF1 associated skeletal manifestations such as pseudarthrosis and osteoporosis which carry significant morbidity and are refractory to current modalities.

CONCLUSION

Human tissue and animal models now suggest that heterotypic interactions between multiple cells types with varying NF1 gene dose are central to the pathogenesis of NF1 associated skeletal anomalies. Here we summarize the experimental evidence that *Nf1* haploinsufficient hematopoietic derived myeloid progenitor cells and osteoclasts play a critical role in potentiating osteolytic activity, cooperating with *Nf1* deficient mesenchymal cells and osteoblasts to engender multiple NF1 associated osseous defects including osteoporosis and fracture non-union (pseudarthrosis) in transgenic mouse models of the human disease. Beyond augmenting osteoblast bone anabolic activity, further clinical trials are needed to determine the therapeutic relevance of targeting *NF1* heterozygous osteoclasts and hematopoietic progenitor cells in the treatment of NF1 bone manifestations. In the interim, further exploration of heterotypic cellular interactions within the bone microenvironment will continue to facilitate the identification of novel, targeted therapies to effectively treat NF1 associated skeletal anomalies.

REFERENCES

[1]   Friedman, J; et al., Neurofibromatosis: phenotype, natural history, and pathogenesis. 3rd ed. Baltimore, MD: The Johns Hopkins University Press, 1999.
[2]   Ballester, R; et al., The NF1 locus encodes a protein functionally related to mammalian GAP and yeast IRA proteins. *Cell,* 1990, 63(4), 851-9.
[3]   Xu, GF; et al., The neurofibromatosis type 1 gene encodes a protein related to GAP. *Cell*, 1990, 62(3), 599-608.

[4]   Martin, GA; et al., The GAP-related domain of the neurofibromatosis type 1 gene product interacts with ras p21, *Cell*, 1990, 63(4), 843-9.

[5]   Riccardi, VM; Von Recklinghausen neurofibromatosis. *N Engl J Med*, 1981, 305(27), 1617-27.

[6]   Friedman, JM; Birch, PH. Type 1 neurofibromatosis: a descriptive analysis of the disorder in 1,728 patients. *Am J Med Genet*, 1997, 70(2), 138-43.

[7]   Friedman, JM; Epidemiology of neurofibromatosis type 1, *Am J Med Genet*, 1999, 89(1), 1-6.

[8]   Listernick, R; et al., Optic gliomas in children with neurofibromatosis type 1, *J Pediatr*, 1989, 114(5), 788-92.

[9]   Listernick, R; et al., Natural history of optic pathway tumors in children with neurofibromatosis type 1: a longitudinal study. *J Pediatr*, 1994, 125(1), 63-6.

[10]   Lubs, ML; et al., Lisch nodules in neurofibromatosis type 1, *N Engl J Med*, 1991, 324(18), 1264-6.

[11]   Hyman, SL; Shores, A; North, KN. The nature and frequency of cognitive deficits in children with neurofibromatosis type 1, *Neurology*, 2005, 65(7), 1037-44.

[12]   Lin, AE; et al., Cardiovascular malformations and other cardiovascular abnormalities in neurofibromatosis 1, *Am J Med Genet*, 2000, 95(2), 108-17.

[13]   Fossali, E; et al., Renovascular disease and hypertension in children with neurofibromatosis. *Pediatr Nephrol*, 2000, 14(8-9), 806-10.

[14]   Rasmussen, SA; Yang, Q; Friedman, JM. Mortality in neurofibromatosis 1: an analysis using U.S. death certificates. *Am J Hum Genet*, 2001, 68(5), 1110-8.

[15]   Friedman, JM; et al., Cardiovascular disease in neurofibromatosis 1: report of the NF1 Cardiovascular Task Force. *Genet Med*, 2002, 4(3), 105-11.

[16]   Lama, G; et al., Blood pressure and cardiovascular involvement in children with neurofibromatosis type1, *Pediatr Nephrol*, 2004, 19(4), 413-8.

[17]   Rea, D; et al., Cerebral arteriopathy in children with neurofibromatosis type 1, *Pediatrics*, 2009, 124(3), e476-83.

[18]   Brodeur, GM. The NF1 gene in myelopoiesis and childhood myelodysplastic syndromes. *N Engl J Med*, 1994, 330(9), 637-9.

[19] Side, L; et al., Homozygous inactivation of the NF1 gene in bone marrow cells from children with neurofibromatosis type 1 and malignant myeloid disorders. *N Engl J Med*, 1997, 336(24), 1713-20.

[20] Emanuel, PD; et al., The role of monocyte-derived hemopoietic growth factors in the regulation of myeloproliferation in juvenile chronic myelogenous leukemia. *Exp Hematol*, 1991, 19(10), 1017-24.

[21] Lammert, M; et al., Decreased bone mineral density in patients with neurofibromatosis 1, *Osteoporos Int*, 2005, 16(9), 1161-6.

[22] Kuorilehto, T; et al., Decreased bone mineral density and content in neurofibromatosis type 1: lowest local values are located in the load-carrying parts of the body. *Osteoporos Int*, 2005, 16(8), 928-36.

[23] Dulai, S; et al., Decreased bone mineral density in neurofibromatosis type 1: results from a pediatric cohort. *J Pediatr Orthop*, 2007, 27(4), 472-5.

[24] Yilmaz, K; et al., Bone mineral density in children with neurofibromatosis 1, *Acta Paediatr*, 2007, 96(8), 1220-2.

[25] Stevenson, DA; et al., Bone mineral density in children and adolescents with neurofibromatosis type 1, *J Pediatr*, 2007, 150(1), 83-8.

[26] Tucker, T; et al., Bone health and fracture rate in individuals with neurofibromatosis 1 (NF1). *J Med Genet*, 2009, 46(4), 259-65.

[27] Crawford, AH. Pitfalls of spinal deformities associated with neurofibromatosis in children. *Clin Orthop Relat Res*, 1989(245), 29-42.

[28] Crawford, AH; Jr; N. Bagamery, Osseous manifestations of neurofibromatosis in childhood. *J Pediatr Orthop*, 1986, 6(1), 72-88.

[29] Illes, T; et al., Decreased bone mineral density in neurofibromatosis-1 patients with spinal deformities. *Osteoporos Int*, 2001, 12(10), 823-7.

[30] Clementi, M; et al., Neurofibromatosis type 1 growth charts. *Am J Med Genet*, 1999, 87(4), 317-23.

[31] Szudek, J; Birch, P; Friedman, JM. Growth in North American white children with neurofibromatosis 1 (NF1). *J Med Genet*, 2000, 37(12), 933-8.

[32] Virdis, R; et al., Growth and pubertal disorders in neurofibromatosis type 1, *J Pediatr Endocrinol Metab*, 2003, 16 Suppl 2: p. 289-92.

[33] Riccardi, VM. Neurofibromatosis : phenotype, natural history, and pathogenesis. 2nd ed. 1992, Baltimore: Johns Hopkins University Press. ix, 498 p.

[34] Alwan, S., Tredwell, SJ; Friedman, JM. Is osseous dysplasia a primary feature of neurofibromatosis 1 (NF1)? *Clin Genet*, 2005, 67(5), 378-90.

[35] Elefteriou, F; et al., Skeletal abnormalities in neurofibromatosis type 1: approaches to therapeutic options. *Am J Med Genet A*, 2009, 149A(10), 2327-38.

[36] Young, H; Hyman, S; North, K. Neurofibromatosis 1: clinical review and exceptions to the rules. *J Child Neurol*, 2002, 17(8), 613-21; discussion 627-9, 646-51.

[37] Friedman, JM. Neurofibromatosis 1: clinical manifestations and diagnostic criteria. *J Child Neurol*, 2002, 17(8), 548-54; discussion 571-2, 646-51.

[38] Stevenson, DA; et al., Descriptive analysis of tibial pseudarthrosis in patients with neurofibromatosis 1, *Am J Med Genet*, 1999, 84(5), 413-9.

[39] Rosen, HN; et al., Specificity of urinary excretion of cross-linked N-telopeptides of type I collagen as a marker of bone turnover. *Calcif Tissue Int*, 1994, 54(1), 26-9.

[40] Delmas, PD; et al., Urinary excretion of pyridinoline crosslinks correlates with bone turnover measured on iliac crest biopsy in patients with vertebral osteoporosis. *J Bone Miner Res*, 1991, 6(6), 639-44.

[41] Robins, SP; et al., Evaluation of urinary hydroxypyridinium crosslink measurements as resorption markers in metabolic bone diseases. *Eur J Clin Invest*, 1991, 21(3), 310-5.

[42] Stevenson, DA; et al., Evidence of increased bone resorption in neurofibromatosis type 1 using urinary pyridinium crosslink analysis. *Pediatr Res*, 2008, 63(6), 697-701.

[43] Heerva, E; et al., A controlled register based study of 460 neurofibromatosis 1 (NF1) patients: Increased fracture risk in children and adults over 41 years. *J Bone Miner Res*, 2012.

[44] Gould, E. The bone changes occuring in Von Recklinghausen's disease. *Q J Med*, 1918, 11, 221-228.

[45] Weiss, R. (A) Von Recklinghausen's disease in the Negro; (B) curvature of the spine in von Recklinghausen's disease. *Arch Dermatol Syphilol*, 1921, 3, 144-151.

[46] Akbarnia, BA; et al., Prevalence of scoliosis in neurofibromatosis. *Spine* (Phila Pa 1976), 1992, 17(8 Suppl), S244-8.

[47] Rezaian, SM., The incidence of scoliosis due to neurofibromatosis. *Acta Orthop Scand*, 1976, 47(5), 534-9.

[48] Tsirikos, AI; et al., Assessment of vertebral scalloping in neurofibromatosis type 1 with plain radiography and MRI. *Clin Radiol*, 2004, 59(11), 1009-17.

[49] Vitale, MG; Guha, A; Skaggs, DL. Orthopaedic manifestations of neurofibromatosis in children: an update. *Clin Orthop Relat Res*, 2002(401), 107-18.

[50] Durrani, AA; et al., Modulation of spinal deformities in patients with neurofibromatosis type 1, *Spine* (Phila Pa 1976), 2000, 25(1), 69-75.

[51] Abdel-Wanis, ME; Kawahara, N. The role of neurofibromin and melatonin in pathogenesis of pseudarthrosis after spinal fusion for neurofibromatous scoliosis. *Med Hypotheses*, 2002, 58(5), 395-8.

[52] Xu, M; et al., Constitutive mobilization of CD34+ cells into the peripheral blood in idiopathic myelofibrosis may be due to the action of a number of proteases. *Blood*, 2005, 105(11), 4508-15.

[53] Kim, HW; Weinstein, SL. Spine update. The management of scoliosis in neurofibromatosis. *Spine* (Phila Pa 1976), 1997, 22(23), 2770-6.

[54] Peltier, LF. The classic. Ununited fractures in children. James Paget, 1891, *Clin Orthop Relat Res*, 1982(166), 2-4.

[55] Delgado-Martinez, AD; Rodriguez-Merchan, EC; Olsen, B. Congenital pseudarthrosis of the tibia. *Int Orthop*, 1996, 20(3), 192-9.

[56] Sofield, HA., Congenital pseudarthrosis of the tibia. *Clin Orthop Relat Res*, 1971, 76, 33-42.

[57] Morrissy, RT; Riseborough, EJ; Hall, JE. Congenital pseudarthrosis of the tibia. *J Bone Joint Surg Br*, 1981, 63-B(3), 367-75.

[58] Gilbert, A; Brockman, R. Congenital pseudarthrosis of the tibia. Long-term followup of 29 cases treated by microvascular bone transfer. *Clin Orthop Relat Res*, 1995, (314), 37-44.

[59] Ippolito, E; et al., Pathology of bone lesions associated with congenital pseudarthrosis of the leg. J Pediatr Orthop B, 2000, 9(1), 3-10.

[60] Cho, TJ; et al., Biologic characteristics of fibrous hamartoma from congenital pseudarthrosis of the tibia associated with neurofibromatosis type 1, *J Bone Joint Surg Am*, 2008, 90(12), 2735-44.

[61] Boyd, HB., Pathology and natural history of congenital pseudarthrosis of the tibia. *Clin Orthop Relat Res*, 1982(166), 5-13.

[62] Leskela, HV; et al., Congenital pseudarthrosis of neurofibromatosis type 1: impaired osteoblast differentiation and function and altered NF1 gene expression. *Bone*, 2009, 44(2), 243-50.

[63] Calvi, LM; et al., Osteoblastic cells regulate the haematopoietic stem cell niche. *Nature*, 2003, 425(6960), 841-6.

[64] Nilsson, SK; et al., Osteopontin, a key component of the hematopoietic stem cell niche and regulator of primitive hematopoietic progenitor cells. *Blood*, 2005, 106(4), 1232-9.

[65] Stier, S; et al., Osteopontin is a hematopoietic stem cell niche component that negatively regulates stem cell pool size. *J Exp Med*, 2005, 201(11), 1781-91.

[66] Zhang, J; et al., Identification of the haematopoietic stem cell niche and control of the niche size. *Nature*, 2003, 425(6960), 836-41.

[67] Arai, F; et al., Tie2/angiopoietin-1 signaling regulates hematopoietic stem cell quiescence in the bone marrow niche. *Cell*, 2004, 118(2), 149-61.

[68] Taichman, RS; Reilly, MJ; Emerson, SG. The Hematopoietic Microenvironment: Osteoblasts and The Hematopoietic Microenvironment. *Hematology*, 2000, 4(5), 421-426.

[69] Mayack, SR; Wagers, AJ. Osteolineage niche cells initiate hematopoietic stem cell mobilization. *Blood*, 2008, 112(3), 519-31.

[70] Orkin, SH; Zon, LI. Hematopoiesis: an evolving paradigm for stem cell biology. *Cell*, 2008, 132(4), 631-44.

[71] Yoshida, H; et al., The murine mutation osteopetrosis is in the coding region of the macrophage colony stimulating factor gene. *Nature*, 1990, 345(6274), 442-4.

[72] Lacey, DL; et al., Osteoprotegerin ligand is a cytokine that regulates osteoclast differentiation and activation. *Cell*, 1998, 93(2), 165-76.

[73] Yasuda, H; et al., Osteoclast differentiation factor is a ligand for osteoprotegerin/osteoclastogenesis-inhibitory factor and is identical to TRANCE/RANKL. *Proc Natl Acad Sci U S A*, 1998, 95(7), 3597-602.

[74] Novack, DV; Teitelbaum, SL. The osteoclast: friend or foe? *Annu Rev Pathol*, 2008, 3: p. 457-84.

[75] Lomaga, MA; et al., TRAF6 deficiency results in osteopetrosis and defective interleukin-1, CD40, and LPS signaling. *Genes Dev*, 1999, 13(8), 1015-24.

[76] Marks, SC; Jr. Seifert, MF; McGuire, JL. Congenitally osteopetrotic (oplop) mice are not cured by transplants of spleen or bone marrow cells from normal littermates. *Metab Bone Dis Relat Res*, 1984, 5(4), 183-6.

[77] Kong, YY; et al., OPGL is a key regulator of osteoclastogenesis, lymphocyte development and lymph-node organogenesis. *Nature*, 1999, 397(6717), 315-23.

[78] Li, J; et al., RANK is the intrinsic hematopoietic cell surface receptor that controls osteoclastogenesis and regulation of bone mass and calcium metabolism. *Proc Natl Acad Sci U S A*, 2000, 97(4), 1566-71.

[79] Coccia, PF; et al., Successful bone-marrow transplantation for infantile malignant osteopetrosis. *N Engl J Med*, 1980, 302(13), 701-8.

[80] Bucay, N; et al., osteoprotegerin-deficient mice develop early onset osteoporosis and arterial calcification. *Genes Dev*, 1998, 12(9), 1260-8.

[81] Damen, JE; et al., The 145-kDa protein induced to associate with Shc by multiple cytokines is an inositol tetraphosphate and phosphatidylinositol 3,4,5-triphosphate 5-phosphatase. *Proc Natl Acad Sci U S A*, 1996, 93(4), 1689-93.

[82] Huber, M; et al., The src homology 2-containing inositol phosphatase (SHIP) is the gatekeeper of mast cell degranulation. *Proc Natl Acad Sci U S A*, 1998, 95(19), 11330-5.

[83] Takeshita, S; et al., SHIP-deficient mice are severely osteoporotic due to increased numbers of hyper-resorptive osteoclasts. *Nat Med*, 2002, 8(9), 943-9.

[84] Silberstein, R; et al., Bone remodeling in W/Wv mast cell deficient mice. *Bone*, 1991, 12(4), 227-36.

[85] Fitzpatrick, LA; et al., Targeted deletion of histidine decarboxylase gene in mice increases bone formation and protects against ovariectomy-induced bone loss. *Proc Natl Acad Sci U S A*, 2003, 100(10), 6027-32.

[86] Dobigny, C; Saffar, JL. H1 and H2 histamine receptors modulate osteoclastic resorption by different pathways: evidence obtained by using receptor antagonists in a rat synchronized resorption model. *J Cell Physiol*, 1997, 173(1), 10-8.

[87] Lesclous, P; et al., Histamine participates in the early phase of trabecular bone loss in ovariectomized rats. *Bone*, 2004, 34(1), 91-9.

[88] Fallon, MD; Whyte, MP; Teitelbaum, SL. Systemic mastocytosis associated with generalized osteopenia. Histopathological characterization of the skeletal lesion using undecalcified bone from two patients. *Hum Pathol*, 1981, 12(9), 813-20.

[89] Theoharides, TC; Boucher, W; Spear, K. Serum interleukin-6 reflects disease severity and osteoporosis in mastocytosis patients. *Int Arch Allergy Immunol*, 2002, 128(4), 344-50.

[90] McDaniel, AS; et al., Pak1 regulates multiple c-Kit mediated Ras-MAPK gain-in-function phenotypes in Nf1+/- mast cells. *Blood*, 2008, 112(12), 4646-54.

[91] Horowitz, MC; Fretz, JA; Lorenzo, JA. How B cells influence bone biology in health and disease. *Bone*, 2010, 47(3), 472-9.

[92] Pacifici, R. T cells: critical bone regulators in health and disease. *Bone*, 2010, 47(3), 461-71.

[93] Kacena, MA; Gundberg, CM; Horowitz, MC. A reciprocal regulatory interaction between megakaryocytes, bone cells, and hematopoietic stem cells. *Bone*, 2006, 39(5), 978-84.

[94] Kacena, MA; Horowitz, MC. The role of megakaryocytes in skeletal homeostasis and rheumatoid arthritis. *Curr Opin Rheumatol*, 2006, 18(4), 405-10.

[95] Rodan, GA; Martin, TJ. Role of osteoblasts in hormonal control of bone resorption--a hypothesis. *Calcif Tissue Int*, 1981, 33(4), 349-51.

[96] Wiktor-Jedrzejczak, W; et al., Total absence of colony-stimulating factor 1 in the macrophage-deficient osteopetrotic (op/op) mouse. *Proc Natl Acad Sci U S A*, 1990, 87(12), 4828-32.

[97] Simonet, WS; et al., Osteoprotegerin: a novel secreted protein involved in the regulation of bone density. *Cell*, 1997, 89(2), 309-19.

[98] Graves, DT; Jiang, Y; Valente, AJ. The expression of monocyte chemoattractant protein-1 and other chemokines by osteoblasts. *Front Biosci*, 1999, 4, p. D571-80.

[99] Chellaiah, MA; Hruska, KA. The integrin alpha(v)beta(3) and CD44 regulate the actions of osteopontin on osteoclast motility. *Calcif Tissue Int*, 2003, 72(3), 197-205.

[100] Li, H; et al., Ras dependent paracrine secretion of osteopontin by Nf1+/- osteoblasts promote osteoclast activation in a neurofibromatosis type I murine model. *Pediatr Res*, 2009, 65(6), 613-8.

[101] Elefteriou, F; et al., ATF4 mediation of NF1 functions in osteoblast reveals a nutritional basis for congenital skeletal dysplasiae. *Cell Metab*, 2006, 4(6), 441-51.

[102] Tang, Y; et al., TGF-beta1-induced migration of bone mesenchymal stem cells couples bone resorption with formation. *Nat Med*, 2009, 15(7), 757-65.

[103] Loeys, BL; et al., A syndrome of altered cardiovascular, craniofacial, neurocognitive and skeletal development caused by mutations in TGFBR1 or TGFBR2, *Nat Genet*, 2005, 37(3), 275-81.

[104] Kirmani, S; et al., Germline TGF-beta receptor mutations and skeletal fragility: a report on two patients with Loeys-Dietz syndrome. *Am J Med Genet A*, 2010, 152A(4), 1016-9.

[105] Ben Amor, IM; et al., Low bone mass and high material bone density in two patients with Loeys-Dietz syndrome caused by transforming growth factor receptor 2 mutations. *J Bone Miner Res*, 2011.

[106] Sousa, SB; et al., Expanding the skeletal phenotype of Loeys-Dietz syndrome. *Am J Med Genet A*, 2011, 155A(5), 1178-83.

[107] Wilner, HI; N. Finby, Skeletal Manifestations in the Marfan Syndrome. *JAMA*, 1964, 187: p. 490-5.

[108] Kohlmeier, L; et al., The bone mineral status of patients with Marfan syndrome. *J Bone Miner Res*, 1995, 10(10), 1550-5.

[109] Le Parc, JM; et al., Bone mineral density in sixty adult patients with Marfan syndrome. *Osteoporos Int*, 1999, 10(6), 475-9.

[110] Moura, B; et al., Bone mineral density in Marfan syndrome. A large case-control study. *Joint Bone Spine*, 2006, 73(6), 733-5.

[111] Demetracopoulos, CA; Sponseller, PD. Spinal deformities in Marfan syndrome. *Orthop Clin North Am*, 2007, 38(4), 563-72, vii.

[112] Janssens, K; et al., Camurati-Engelmann disease: review of the clinical, radiological, and molecular data of 24 families and implications for diagnosis and treatment. *J Med Genet*, 2006, 43(1), 1-11.

[113] Rhodes, SD; et al., Hyperactive transforming growth factor-beta1 signaling potentiates skeletal defects in a neurofibromatosis type 1 mouse model. *J Bone Miner Res*, 2013, 28(12), 2476-89.

[114] Zhao, C; et al., Bidirectional ephrinB2-EphB4 signaling controls bone homeostasis. *Cell Metab*, 2006, 4(2), 111-21.

[115] Negishi-Koga, T; et al., Suppression of bone formation by osteoclastic expression of semaphorin 4D. *Nat Med*, 2011, 17(11), 1473-80.

[116] Largaespada, DA; et al., Nf1 deficiency causes Ras-mediated granulocyte/macrophage colony stimulating factor hypersensitivity and chronic myeloid leukaemia. *Nat Genet*, 1996, 12(2), 137-43.

[117] Bollag, G; et al., Loss of NF1 results in activation of the Ras signaling pathway and leads to aberrant growth in haematopoietic cells. *Nat Genet*, 1996, 12(2), 144-8.

[118] Zhang, Y; et al., Quantitative effects of Nf1 inactivation on in vivo hematopoiesis. *J Clin Invest*, 2001, 108(5), 709-15.

[119] Ingram, DA; et al., Leukemic potential of doubly mutant Nf1 and Wv hematopoietic cells. *Blood*, 2003, 101(5), 1984-6.

[120] Zhang, YY; et al., Nf1 regulates hematopoietic progenitor cell growth and ras signaling in response to multiple cytokines. *J Exp Med*, 1998, 187(11), 1893-902.

[121] Staser, K; et al., Normal hematopoiesis and neurofibromin-deficient myeloproliferative disease require Erk. *J Clin Invest*, 2013, 123(1), 329-34.

[122] Chang, T; et al., Sustained MEK inhibition abrogates myeloproliferative disease in Nf1 mutant mice. *J Clin Invest*, 2013, 123(1), 335-9.

[123] Yang, FC; et al., Nf1-dependent tumors require a microenvironment containing Nf1+/-- and c-kit-dependent bone marrow. *Cell*, 2008, 135(3), 437-48.

[124] Lasater, EA; et al., Genetic and cellular evidence of vascular inflammation in neurofibromin-deficient mice and humans. *J Clin Invest*, 2010, 120(3), 859-70.

[125] Stansfield, BK; et al., Heterozygous inactivation of the Nf1 gene in myeloid cells enhances neointima formation via a rosuvastatin-sensitive cellular pathway. *Hum Mol Genet*, 2013, 22(5), 977-88.

[126] Lakkis, MM; Epstein, JA. Neurofibromin modulation of ras activity is required for normal endocardial-mesenchymal transformation in the developing heart. *Development*, 1998, 125(22), 4359-67.

[127] Yang, FC; et al., Hyperactivation of p21ras and PI3K cooperate to alter murine and human neurofibromatosis type 1-haploinsufficient osteoclast functions. *J Clin Invest*, 2006, 116(11), 2880-91.

[128] Heerva, E; et al., Osteoclasts in neurofibromatosis type 1 display enhanced resorption capacity, aberrant morphology, and resistance to serum deprivation. *Bone*, 2010, 47(3), 583-90.

[129] Stevenson, DA; et al., Multiple increased osteoclast functions in individuals with neurofibromatosis type 1, *Am J Med Genet A*, 2011, 155A(5), 1050-9.

[130] Yan, J; et al., Rac1 mediates the osteoclast gains-in-function induced by haploinsufficiency of Nf1, *Hum Mol Genet*, 2008, 17(7), 936-48.

[131] He, Y; et al., Erk1 positively regulates osteoclast differentiation and bone resorptive activity. *PLoS One*, 2011, 6(9), e24780.

[132] Saulnier, N; et al., ERK1 regulates the hematopoietic stem cell niches. *PLoS One*, 2012, 7(1), e30788.

[133] Wu, X; et al., Neurofibromin plays a critical role in modulating osteoblast differentiation of mesenchymal stem/progenitor cells. *Hum Mol Genet*, 2006, 15(19), 2837-45.

[134] Yu, X; et al., Neurofibromin and its inactivation of Ras are prerequisites for osteoblast functioning. *Bone*, 2005, 36(5), 793-802.

[135] Schindeler, A; et al., Models of tibial fracture healing in normal and Nf1-deficient mice. *J Orthop Res*, 2008, 26(8), 1053-60.

[136] Wang, W; et al., Local low-dose lovastatin delivery improves the bone-healing defect caused by Nf1 loss of function in osteoblasts. *J Bone Miner Res*, 2010, 25(7), 1658-67.

[137] Stevenson, DA; et al., Double inactivation of NF1 in tibial pseudarthrosis. *Am J Hum Genet*, 2006, 79(1), 143-8.

[138] Lee, SM; et al., Is double inactivation of the Nf1 gene responsible for the development of congenital pseudarthrosis of the tibia associated with NF1? *J Orthop Res*, 2012.

[139] Wu, X; et al., The haploinsufficient hematopoietic microenvironment is critical to the pathological fracture repair in murine models of neurofibromatosis type 1, *PLoS One*, 2011, 6(9), e24917.

[140] Zhang, W; et al., Primary osteopathy of vertebrae in a neurofibromatosis type 1 murine model. *Bone*, 2011, 48(6), 1378-87.

[141] Kolanczyk, M; et al., Multiple roles for neurofibromin in skeletal development and growth. *Hum Mol Genet*, 2007, 16(8), 874-86.

[142] Wang, W; et al., Mice lacking Nf1 in osteochondroprogenitor cells display skeletal dysplasia similar to patients with neurofibromatosis type I. *Hum Mol Genet*, 2011, 20(20), 3910-24.

[143] Alanne, MH; et al., Phenotypic characterization of transgenic mice harboring Nf1(+/-) or Nf1(-/-) osteoclasts in otherwise Nf1(+/+) background. *J Cell Biochem*, 2012.

[144] Chiu, WS; et al., Transgenic mice that express Cre recombinase in osteoclasts. *Genesis*, 2004, 39(3), 178-85.

[145] Clausen, BE; et al., Conditional gene targeting in macrophages and granulocytes using LysMcre mice. *Transgenic Res*, 1999, 8(4), 265-77.

[146] El-Hoss, J; et al., A murine model of neurofibromatosis type 1 tibial pseudarthrosis featuring proliferative fibrous tissue and osteoclast-like cells. *J Bone Miner Res*, 2011.

[147] Xu, XL; et al., Basic research and clinical applications of bisphosphonates in bone disease: what have we learned over the last 40 years? *J Transl Med*, 2013, 11, p. 303.

[148] Heerva, E; et al., Osteoclasts derived from patients with neurofibromatosis 1 (NF1) display insensitivity to bisphosphonates in vitro. *Bone*, 2012, 50(3), 798-803.

[149] Heerva, E; et al., Follow-up of six patients with neurofibromatosis 1-related osteoporosis treated with alendronate for 23 months. *Calcif Tissue Int*, 2014, 94(6), 608-12.

[150] Seitz, S; et al., High bone turnover and accumulation of osteoid in patients with neurofibromatosis 1, *Osteoporos Int*, 2010, 21(1), 119-27.

[151] Brunetti-Pierri, N; et al., Generalized metabolic bone disease in Neurofibromatosis type I. *Mol Genet Metab*, 2008, 94(1), 105-11.

[152] He, Y; et al., c-Fms signaling mediates neurofibromatosis Type-1 osteoclast gain-in-functions. *PLoS One*, 2012, 7(11), e46900.

[153] Birke, O; et al., Preliminary experience with the combined use of recombinant bone morphogenetic protein and bisphosphonates in the treatment of congenital pseudarthrosis of the tibia. *J Child Orthop*, 2010, 4(6), 507-17.

[154] Schindeler, A; et al., Distal tibial fracture repair in a neurofibromatosis type 1-deficient mouse treated with recombinant bone morphogenetic protein and a bisphosphonate. *J Bone Joint Surg Br*, 2011, 93(8), 1134-9.

[155] Kolanczyk, M; et al., Modelling neurofibromatosis type 1 tibial dysplasia and its treatment with lovastatin. *BMC Med*, 2008, 6, p. 21.

[156] Sharma, R; et al., Hyperactive Ras/MAPK signaling is critical for tibial nonunion fracture in neurofibromin-deficient mice. *Hum Mol Genet*, 2013, 22(23), 4818-28.

[157] El-Hoss, J; et al., A Combination of rhBMP-2 (Recombinant Human Bone Morphogenetic Protein-2) and MEK (MAP Kinase/ERK Kinase) Inhibitor PD0325901 Increases Bone Formation in a Murine Model of Neurofibromatosis Type I Pseudarthrosis. *J Bone Joint Surg Am*, 2014, 96(14), e117.

[158] de la Croix Ndong, J; et al., Asfotase-alpha improves bone growth, mineralization and strength in mouse models of neurofibromatosis type-1, *Nat Med*, 2014, 20(8), 904-10.

In: Neurofibromatosis
Editor: Walter Romaine

ISBN: 978-1-63463-229-4
© 2015 Nova Science Publishers, Inc.

Chapter 3

CEREBROVASCULAR COMPLICATIONS OF NEUROFIBROMATOSIS TYPE I

*Patrick M. Flanigan[1] and Richard A. Prayson[1,2]**
[1]Cleveland Clinic Lerner College of Medicine of Case
Western Reserve University, Ohio, US
[2]Cleveland Clinic Department of Pathology, Ohio, US

ABSTRACT

Neurofibromatosis Type 1 (NF1) is a hereditary neurocutaneous tumor disorder that owes many of its most common features to abnormalities in neural crest-derived cells. NF1 may cause dysplasia in various tissues, even in some tissues that are non-neural crest-derived (e.g. bone). While common manifestations of NF1 include café-au-lait spots and neurofibromas, vasculopathies are less common yet noteworthy complications of NF1. NF1 vasculopathies can involve vessels supplying various organs. Cerebrovascular abnormalities associated with NF1 have been sporadically described in the literature; these conditions are of interest due to the incomplete understanding of their pathogenesis and genetics.

NF1 is associated with a diverse set of cerebrovascular complications including stenosis/occlusive disease, aneurysm, arteriovenous malformations, Moya Moya disease, arteriovenous fistulas, spontaneous

* Correspondence: Richard Prayson, MD, Department of Pathology, L25, Cleveland Clinic, 9500 Euclid Avenue, Cleveland, Ohio 44195 USA, Phone: 216-444-8805, FAX: 216-445-6967, Email: praysor@ccf.org.

vascular rupture, and arteries compressed or invaded by neural tumors. The most common cerebrovascular abnormality in NF1 patients is occlusion or stenosis of the cerebral arteries. In this chapter, we describe the cerebrovascular complications of NF1 focusing on the pathology of the aforementioned subtypes, pathogenesis, clinical features, outcomes, proposed therapies and genetics.

INTRODUCTION

Neurofibromatosis Type 1 (NF1) is a primary neurocutaneous syndrome [1, 2], sometimes referred to as von Recklinghausen disease type 1. NF1 is an autosomal dominant disorder with pathologies resulting from the maldevelopment of neural crest cells, although non-neural crest-derived tissues are also affected [3–5]. The syndrome exhibits near 100% penetrance with marked variability in its expressivity even within families [6]. NF1 is sometimes considered a syndrome rather than a disease as its exact etiology is not completely delineated. NF1 is associated with a loss-of-function mutation of a tumor suppressor gene called neurofibromin, an inhibitor of p21 ras oncoprotein, on chromosome 17 [4, 5]. Overactivity of ras is thought to cause some of the manifestations of NF1. In more than 95% of individuals with NF1, a mutation has been identified with about 50% of individuals having an affected parent and 50% having the altered gene as a result of de novo (e.g. germline) mutation [7]. Over 500 mutations in the NF1 gene have been identified, most being unique to each family [7].

As mentioned, overactivity of ras may cause some of the manifestations of NF1 and some ras-independent mechanisms of neurofibromin have been proposed (e.g. regulation of adenylyl cyclase activity) [8]. More specifically, neurofibromin is an activator of ras GTPase, which hydrolyzes active ras-GTP to inactive ras-GDP [9]. Reduction or complete loss of neurofibromin activity thereby leads to activation of ras via decreased inhibition. Ras regulates many downstream signaling pathways (e.g. mitogen-activated protein kinase (MAPK), phosphatidylinositol 3-kinase (PI3K), protein kinase B (PKB), and mammalian target of rapamycin (mTOR) kinase). The net result of mutations in neurofibromin is activation of the aforementioned pathways which stimulate cellular proliferation and survival (among other cellular effects) [10]. Neurofibromin expression has been found in both smooth muscle and endothelial cells of blood vessels [8].

NF1 typically involves dysplasia of the soft tissue, central and peripheral nervous system, and skin and is characterized by multiple café-au-lait macules, subcutaneous or cutaneous neurofibromas, optic gliomas, axillary and inguinal freckling, and iris Lisch nodules (hamartomas) [11, 12]. While these findings are among the most common, the manifestations of NF1 vary from patient to patient (even among families) and dysplasia in other tissues such as bone, endocrine organs, and blood vessels also occurs in some individuals [13]. The average life expectancy of patients with NF1 is eight to15 years less than the average person [14–16]. Relatedly, malignant peripheral nerve sheath tumors and vasculopathy are the two most important pathologies that contribute to early death in individuals with NF1 [4]. Indeed, despite their relative rarity, intrinsic vasculopathies and vascular impairment due to extrinsic factors (e.g. arterial compression by tumors) in NF1 have important and sometimes devastating clinical consequences [17, 18]; these are the focus of this review chapter.

NF1 VASCULOPATHIES OVERVIEW

The diversity of ways in which the vasculature can be disrupted in NF1 is myriad and evidenced by the numerous unique cases that have been outlined in the literature [17, 19–26]. Despite the diversity of presentations and pathologies among different patients, some general trends in vasculopathies are worth noting. A majority of the patients with NF1 and abnormal vasculature have asymptomatic involvement of multiple blood vessels in different organs [3, 27, 28]. Because of this, the exact prevalence of vascular lesions in NF1 patients is hard to determine; however, large clinical series have reported a prevalence anywhere from 0.4% to 6.4% [3, 17, 27–29]. More recent studies suggest that prevalence of these lesions may have been previously underestimated because new imaging techniques (magnetic resonance angiography) are superior in their detection of vascular abnormalities in NF1 patients [30, 31]. When symptoms do manifest, they usually occur in childhood or early adulthood except in certain less common subtypes of NF1 vasculopathy (e.g. aneurysms and arteriovenous fistulas) [3], [27, 28]. NF1 vasculopathy can affect arterial and venous vessels of any size, although venous involvement is less common than arterial [27, 30]. The most common type of vasculopathy is arterial stenosis, which sometimes leads to eventual arterial occlusion. The renal artery is the vessel most frequently involved, typically resulting in the presentation of renovascular hypertension

[32, 33]. Interestingly, some of the NF1-associated vascular pathologies exhibit different characteristics than they do in patients without the disease. For example, atherosclerotic sites in non-NF1patients tend to occur at the origin or bifurcation of large arteries; whereas, this is not the case for sites of vascular lesions in NF1 patients [17]. Furthermore, vascular lesions in NF1 have been described in virtually all arteries in the human body including in the vasculature of the endocrine system, gastrointestinal tract, heart, and cerebrum [32–34].

In NF1, the cerebral vessels tend to demonstrate the same pathologies as abnormal vessels elsewhere in NF1 patients [26]. While disruptions in the vasculature from invasion or compression of the arterial walls by adjacent neurofibroma(s) does occur and will be discussed later, the typical and more common vasculopathy results from an intrinsic process involving blood vessel walls, which manifests independently from neurofibromas [3, 17, 26]. The genesis of these NF1 vasculopathies is thought to result from an abnormal proliferation in the cells which comprise the blood vessel wall.

In 1944, Reubi [35] was the first to characterize the pathohistology of NF1 vasculopathy. He classified the vascular histology into the purely intimal forms, fusocellular (nodular) forms, and intimal-aneurysmal forms [3, 17, 26]. The purely intimal form is most common and occurs in small arteries 50-400 μm in diameter; this subtype shows a concentric intimal proliferation of spindle cells and thinned media which tends to lead to occlusion of the vascular lumen [36–38]. The fusocellular form occurs in arteries 100-700 μm in diameter; this subtype is characterized by nodular growth of epithelioid or spindle cells in the media or throughout the arterial wall which tends to compromise the strength and integrity of the vessel wall [37, 38]. The intimal-aneurysmal form occurs in arteries 0.5-1 mm in diameter and exhibits eccentric, fibrous intimal proliferation, sparsely distributed spindle cells in the intima and media, fragmentation of elastic tissue, and smooth muscle fibrosis causing aneurysmal dilatation of the vessel wall [37, 38]. Later, two more histological vasculopathies were described -- an epithelioid form and an advanced intimal form. The epithelioid form is characterized by eccentric, fibrous intimal thickening and the advanced intimal form is marked by small aggregates of intimal spindle cells accompanied by a pure intimal form [37]. A finding common to all types is cell accumulation in the intima of the blood vessel [3].

Early work that followed suggested that these proliferating cells were of Schwann-cell origin because of findings of Schwann cell proliferation in the peripheral nervous system of NF1 patients [26]. Subsequent electron microscopy and immunohistochemistry studies demonstrated that the cellular accumulations in the intima were actually of smooth muscle cell origin [3], [26]. A recurring histological finding is fibromuscular dysplasia with marked intimal thickening [3, 17].

This finding is consistent with the identification of neurofibromin expression in smooth muscle cells and endothelial cells of blood vessels [39]. A proposed hypothesis is that neurofibromin plays a role in maintenance of the integrity of the endothelial cell layer and when this role is compromised, the smooth muscle cells are more prone to proliferate [40]. It is well-known that endothelial dysfunction can affect the blood vessel media in several disease processes [41].

For example, in hyaline arteriolosclerosis, chronic hypertension or diabetes mellitus causes endothelial injury, resulting in increased matrix component synthesis by smooth muscle cells. NF1 vasculopathy is believed to be an acquired condition [18].

It has been suggested that NF1 vasculopathy is not an unprovoked dysplastic process resulting from a deficiency in the tumor suppressor gene neurofibromin, but rather the result of an aberration in normal regulation of blood vessel repair and maintenance in which neurofibromin might be implicated [3, 42, 43].

As previously mentioned, the cerebrovasculature exhibits similar pathology to other vessels in NF1, such as intimal thickening and disruption of the internal elastic lamina from the abnormal proliferation of cells of smooth muscle origin. Like other vessels, alteration in cerebral vessel structure often occurs without overt pathophysiological malfunction (i.e. clinically silent)[26]. Furthermore, like renovascular pathology in NF1, cerebrovascular occlusion more frequently arises in the proximal arterial segments as opposed to distal segments [26].

Neurofibromin expression seems to correlate well with the frequency of observed vascular lesions. There is differential expression of neurofibromin in vascular endothelial and smooth muscle cells along the arterial tree which is believed to explain why cerebral and renal vasculature is more frequently affected than the aorta in NF1 vascular dysplasia [8]. Finally, the cerebrovascular lesions in neurofibromatosis display a characteristic distribution in NF1 patients. The supraclinoid (i.e. distal) internal carotid artery is the most frequently involved vessel followed by the middle carotid artery [40]. Posterior cerebral circulation vasculopathy is much less frequent in NF1 patients, accounting for about 10% of the cerebrovasculopathies in NF1 [40, 44]. There are several different categories of cerebrovascular abnormalities in NF1 which are outlined in Table 1. Each of these categories will be discussed in the following sections.

Table 1. Manifestation of cerebrovascular neurofibromatosis

Vascular occlusive disease

    Fibromuscular dysplasia with intimal thickening
    Moya Moya syndrome

Aneurysms

Spontaneous vascular rupture (with or without aneurysm)

Arteriovenous fistula.

Arteries compressed or invaded by neural tumors (neurofibromas including plexiform type, schwannomas, malignant peripheral nerve sheath tumors)

MOYA MOYA SYNDROME AND VASCULAR STENOSIS

Moya Moya syndrome (MMS) is a cerebrovascular condition marked by progressive stenosis of the intracranial internal carotid arteries bilaterally and their branches (e.g. the middle and anterior cerebral arteries) [45–47]. This progressive stenosis results in the concomitant formation of collateral vessels which have a signature "puff of smoke" appearance at the base of the brain on angiography [48]. As a result of MMS, affected individuals are predisposed to develop strokes consequent to progressive narrowing of the intracranial internal carotid arteries.

MMS is a rare condition affecting approximately 1 in 1,000,000 people per year [46]. The incidence of MMS in NF1 far exceeds that of the general population, providing strong evidence for an association. The prevalence of MMS in NF1 patients is estimated to be anywhere between 0.6% and 6% [40], [44, 47, 49]. MMS is believed to account for 47% to 76% of pediatric NF1 cerebrovascular abnormalities [30, 44]. Furthermore, studies have linked one of the genes for hereditary MMS to chromosome 17q25 which is proximal to the NF1 gene on chromosome 17q11.2 [50]. However, because of the relative rarity of MMS and NF1-associated cerebrovasculopathy, the association between these two conditions is not completely understood.

There have been several interesting case reports that attest to the complexity and diversity of the ways in which NF1 patients can be predisposed to develop MMS. In one such case, a patient was receiving bevacizumab for his glioma; gliomas occur more frequently in NF1 patients [51, 52]. Bevacizumab is a promising therapy which targets vascular endothelial growth factor, an important hormone for the angiogenic maintenance of brain tumors. However, because of its intended mechanism of action, bevacizumab can potentially contribute to decreased collateral vessel formation, with consequent reduction of flow and accelerated stenosis of the proximal vasculature [52].

It is estimated that as many as two thirds of patients with MMS experience symptomatic progression over a 5-year period [45]. An interesting area of study has focused on the determination of how NF1 interacts with MMS to change the clinical features (e.g. the progression) of this disease. It is believed that primary MMS and MMS in NF1 patients are comparable clinically, angiographically, and radiographically [48]; however, cranial irradiation is thought to increase the risk of stroke and perioperative complications in MMS patients with NF1 [48]. This again highlights the decreased capacity of NF1 patients to repair their vasculature in an appropriate fashion after a damaging insult, whether endogenous or exogenous.

It is difficult to assess the incidence of stenosis or occlusive disease in NF1, whether isolated or showing a MMS-like pattern, as findings are often incidental [17]. Indeed, most of the occlusive disease associated with NF1 is described as MMS [44]. This is because the stenosis occurs slowly which allows for development of the collateral vessels which are part of the characterization of MMS [20, 47]. However, cases of isolated stenosis and occlusive disease have been occasionally documented in NF1 patients [17].

ANEURYSM

Neurofibromatosis-associated aneurysms in the cerebral vasculature are rare with less than 50 cases being reported in one 2007 review [17]. However, some studies purport that there is increased risk for aneurysms in NF1 patients [53–55]. While many other cerebrovascular lesions associated with NF1 have an average onset in the first two decades of life, the onset of aneurysms in NF1 patients tends to be much later in life [37]. One study found an average age of onset of 40 years for cerebral aneurysms only versus an average age at presentation of 14 years for the onset of occlusive disorders in NF1 patients [37]. NF1-associated aneurysms more commonly occur in the internal carotid artery circulation, and in the anterior communicating and middle cerebral arteries. More rarely, these aneurysms occur in the vertebrobasilar circulation [55]. The distribution pattern of these aneurysms is similar to those found in patients without NF1 [56].

The aneurysms in NF1 patients may be either of the saccular or fusiform variety. The intimal-aneurysmal form of NF1 vasculopathy, as its name implies, is associated with cerebral aneurysms and exhibits eccentric, fibrous intimal proliferation, sparsely distributed spindle cells in the intima and media, fragmentation of elastic tissue and smooth muscle fibrosis [37]. Electron microscopic studies reveal that the spindle cells had smooth muscle cell characteristics with pinocytotic vessels, myofilaments, and electron dense plaques (both free and plasma membrane-bound) [55].

The mechanism of the intrinsic vascular changes that predispose patients to develop aneurysms in NF1 is believed to be similar to mechanisms that underpin the predisposition of normal patients to develop aneurysms – weakening of the supportive connective tissue (e.g. collagen and elastic fibers) and vascular wall smooth muscle [36, 38, 57]. In the setting of NF1 vasculopathy, the weakening of arterial wall is likely secondary to an abnormal proliferation of cells with fibrosis and smooth muscle loss, compromising the structural and functional integrity of the intima and media of the vessel. Interestingly, experimental evidence, using animal models and clinical evidence, suggests that there is aneurysmal vascular pathology associated with proximal arterial obstruction in the setting of NF1 [58, 59]. This evidence suggests that both the formation and growth of the aneurysm is promoted by proximal obstruction of the artery [36].

The fusiform aneurysms are less common than saccular [37, 54]. The fusiform aneurysm is thought to be the result of spontaneous arterial dissection [53]. Fusiform aneurysms tend to occur in the larger cerebral arteries (basilar and internal carotid arteries), typically in a background of atherosclerotic changes [36].

Spontaneous vascular rupture is an extremely rare consequence of NF1 vasculopathy and is usually preceded by aneurysm [29]. In addition, iatrogenic spontaneous vascular ruptures in surgery have been described and are likely a consequence of increased vascular fragility in NF1 patients [29].

ARTERIOVENOUS FISTULAS

Arteriovenous fistulas (AVF) are a rarely encountered form of vasculopathy in NF1. In one 2010 report, there were only 36 known NF1 patients who were afflicted with one or more AVF reported in the literature [60]. Interestingly, the first NF1-associated intracranial AVF was reported in 2008 [61]. The age of onset of NF1-associated AVF is, like aneurysm, much older than age of onset for occlusive NF1 vasculopathy with the average age of onset of AVF in NF1 patients being about 40 years [60, 62]. Also, AVFs and aneurysms are about twice as common in women with NF1 than in men [60, 62].

Generally speaking, the genesis of AVF can be iatrogenic, traumatic, or spontaneous. Spontaneous cases usually arise in vessels with abnormal fragility, such as in the setting of NF1 and other vascular phenomena characterized by fibromuscular dysplasia [63]. In the first report of NF1-associated AVFs, two pathologic mechanisms were proposed [64]. First, it was proposed that compromised structural integrity of the vessel wall from smooth muscle dysplasia or neurofibromatosis predisposes to aneurysm formation which potentiates fistula formation involving the adjacent veins. Alternatively, it has been proposed that the pathogenesis of NF1-associated AVF could be attributed to congenital mesodermal dysplasia. This latter hypothesis is supported by a case of an infant with AVF present from birth who became symptomatic because of heart failure [60].

While AVF in NF1 patients sometimes involves the external carotid artery and occipital artery, the majority of AVF in NF1 patients involve the vertebral artery [62], frequently arising at the V2 and V3 segments of the vertebral artery, which are the most mobile of all vertebral arterial segments. This finding is a testament to the interplay between arterial fragility due to the vascular pathology associated with NF1 and neck mobility in the development of AVF in NF1 patients [62].

ARTERIES COMPRESSED OR INVADED BY NEURAL TUMORS

Neurofibromas, the most common type of tumor associated with NF1, are benign peripheral nerve sheath tumors (PNSTs) which arise from progenitors of Schwann cell origin. Both cutaneous neurofibromas and internal PNSTs are very common in NF1 patients, both occurring individually in over half of individuals. These tumors are embedded in a microenvironment containing perineural cells, mast cells, fibroblasts, and sometimes a highly collagenous extracellular matrix [65]. These benign PNSTs can occur on nerves anywhere in the peripheral nervous system of NF1 patients. Occasionally, plexiform neurofibromas may be seen. These are found almost exclusively in NF1 and are marked by anastomosing cords of neurofibromatous tissue.

This category of tumor-associated vasculopathy in NF1 is distinct from all of the aforementioned vasculopathies associated with NF1 in that it does not result from a pathophysiologic mechanism intrinsic to the blood vessel. Greene et al. divided NF1-associated vascular lesions into two categories [33]. The first category is the previously described intrinsic dysplasia of vessel. The second category involves large arteries (e.g. the carotid artery) that become surrounded by neurofibromatous or ganglioneuromatous tissue. This perivascular involvement by tumor can result in degenerative changes in the vessel wall (e.g. intimal proliferation, fragmentation of the elastic layer, etc.) which can potentiate vascular rupture and aneurysm [44].

Infiltration and compression by tumor predispose NF1 patients to vascular rupture. Leier et al. described two ways in which neurofibromas can potentiate arterial rupture [66]. Neurofibromas can invade the media of the vessel, causing disruption of the vascular smooth muscle thereby reducing the shear strength of the wall. Alternatively, when the vasa vasorum of a large vessel is compressed, this results in ischemia and therefore decreased capacity to support proper synthesis and recycling of matrix elements, thereby weakening the compressed arterial segment [29, 66].

Vascular infiltration and compression by tumors predisposes NF1 patients to aneurysm in both veins and arteries [17]. For example, in a venous aneurysm of the internal jugular vein, neurofibromatous tissue was found in the wall of the aneurysm as well as in the surrounding small veins [63]. The typical finding of myointimal cells in the intima of the arteries, which is characteristic of the mesodermal dysplasia associated with intrinsic NF1 vasculopathy, was not found in the histologic examination of the venous aneurysm. The histologic examination of the wall of the aneurysm showed focal infiltration and partial replacement by neurofibromatous tissue. There were few residual smooth muscle fibers (stained using muscle-specific actin (HHF35)) within the fibrous wall of the aneurysm and a reduction in elastic fibers as well. The adventitia was adherent focally to the neurofibromatous tissue. The hypercellular adventita contained spindle cells and Wagner-Meissner-like bodies were sparse, but present, suggesting involvement of the adventitia by tumor [67]. This study and several others clearly demonstrate that both arterial and venous aneurysms can form as a result of vascular invasion by neurofibromas [17], [67] Neurofibromas, the hallmark of NF1, can give rise to extrinsic vasculopathies interrupting vasculature via compression or infiltration leading to both aneurysms and vascular rupture.

There are three main types of peripheral nerve sheath tumors (neurofibromas, schwannomas, and malignant peripheral nerve sheath tumors) which have different clinical characteristics and treatments. Most of the tumors encountered in the setting of NF1 are neurofibromas. These tumors are derived from cell lineages of the peripheral nerve: perineurial cells, fibroblasts, and Schwann cells [68].

Plexiform neurofibromas are practically pathognomonic for NF1. Neurofibromas typically infiltrate the fascicle of the nerve, are not separable from the nerve, and have poorly defined proximal and distal margins. Microscopically, they have a loose, myxoid stroma with low cellularity; the neurofibroma contains Schwann cells with their ordinary elongated nuclei and extensions of eosinophilic cytoplasm, larger multipolar fibroblastic cells, and a scant amount of inflammatory cells such as mast cells [68]. In contrast, malignant peripheral nerve sheath tumors are more cellular and mitotically active, demonstrate more pronounced cytologic atypia and may contain areas of necrosis. While malignant peripheral nerve sheath tumors, which are larger and more infiltrative by nature, require adjuvant treatment, most benign peripheral nerve sheath tumors require only a simple surgical excision. Currently, there are no approved treatments for NF1-associated plexiform neurofibromas.

Plexiform neurofibromas are resistant to chemoradiotherapy due to their slow-growing rate and cannot be surgically removed due to their frequent proximity to vital body structures (e.g. large arteries). Currently, imatinib mesylate, a tyrosine kinase inhibitor, is being investigated in Phase 2 trials to determine if it can decrease the severity and amount of plexiform neurofibromas in NF1 patients. Imatinib is thought to target mast cells which are important for establishment of the pro-tumor environment possibly necessary for the development of neurofibromas [65].

The preliminary results are somewhat auspicious; six of the 36 patients in the clinical trial showed a 20% or more decrease in tumor volume and minimal adverse reactions to the medication were noted in all patients [69].

OUTCOMES AND PROPOSED APPROACHES TO NF1 VASCULOPATHY

In the literature, surgeons have described vessels of NF1 patients as friable with poor vascular contraction [67]. Because of this, it is believed that NF1-associated arterial dysplasia makes patients more prone to excessive operative hemorrhage [17, 67]. For example, in a report of a surgical repair of a left upper internal jugular venous aneurysm, the patient developed massive hemorrhages [67]. The bleeding was very difficult to control and required two re-explorations and evacuations of cervical hematomas. Due to surgeon's experience with the increased vascular fragility of NF1 patients, carefulness and other operative precautions have been recommended in the literature. For example, when operating on NF1 patients (even without conspicuous vasculopathy), atraumatic, gentle, and delicate handling of tissues, careful placement of retractors, and use of protected, soft arterial clamps during operations is recommended.

Most vascular lesions, including cerebrovascular lesions in NF1 patients, are asymptomatic and discovered incidentally [44]. However, a small proportion of these lesions can later become symptomatic in isolation or be uncovered due to clinical interventions (e.g. surgery, chemotherapy, radiotherapy). Thus, screening of asymptomatic patients poses a clinical dilemma, as many never develop clinically significant symptoms. Currently, there is no definitive consensus in the field on the benefit of screening asymptomatic NF1 patients for vascular abnormalities [17].

From an imaging perspective, magnetic resonance angiography (MRA) allows for superior detection of cerebrovascular abnormalities in NF1 patients. For example, in a recent study in which all patients received MRA of the head, a prevalence of cerebrovascular abnormalities of 7.4% was reported; in 50.0% of the cases, the abnormality was detected by MRA, but not other imaging modalities [47]. As imaging technologies improve, a truer incidence and prevalence of vasculopathy in NF1 patients will likely be determined.

FUTURE DIRECTIONS

Due to the relatively low prevalence of vasculopathies associated with NF1, there remain many opportunities for future investigation. For instance, it has not been completely delineated how other treatments for other pathologies-associated with NF1 interact with vaso-occlusive disease. Antiangiogenesis agents, as previously discussed, may provoke NF1 cerebrovasculopathies, while therapeutic agents currently under investigation (e.g. imatinib) might have a role in delaying the onset or preventing NF1 cerebrovasculopathies [18]. Furthermore, since NF1 is a systemic disorder, associations between different locations and types of vasculopathies could be made. Currently, associations between the co-occurrence of peripheral vascular and cerebrovascular abnormalities is not known. Finally, while MRA is thought to be an effective way to image NF1 vasculopathies, correlation between vascular lesion appearance on imaging and risk of that lesion becoming symptomatic is not currently known, making screening clinically challenging.

REFERENCES

[1]   M. Ruggieri, I. P. Castroviejo, and C. D. Rocco, Neurocutaneous Disorders: Phakomatoses & Hamartoneoplastic Syndromes. Springer, 2009.

[2]   T. Burns, S. Breathnach, N. Cox, and C. Griffiths, Rook's Textbook of Dermatology, 4 Volume Set. John Wiley & Sons, 2010.

[3]   S. J. Hamilton and J. M. Friedman, "Insights into the pathogenesis of neurofibromatosis 1 vasculopathy," *Clin. Genet.*, vol. 58, no. 5, pp. 341–344, Nov. 2000.

[4]   K. Jett and J. M. Friedman, "Clinical and genetic aspects of neurofibromatosis 1," Genet. Med. Off. *J. Am. Coll. Med. Genet.*, vol. 12, no. 1, pp. 1–11, Jan. 2010.

[5]   M. H. Shen, P. S. Harper, and M. Upadhyaya, "Molecular genetics of neurofibromatosis type 1 (NF1)," *J. Med. Genet.,* vol. 33, no. 1, pp. 2–17, Jan. 1996.

[6]   V. M. Riccardi and R. A. Lewis, "Penetrance of von Recklinghausen neurofibromatosis: a distinction between predecessors and descendants.," *Am. J. Hum. Genet.,* vol. 42, no. 2, pp. 284–289, Feb. 1988.

[7]   Genetics in Medicine by Robert L. Nussbaum, MD; Roderick R. McInnes, MD, PhD, FRS(C); and Huntington F. Willard, PhD | eBook on.

[8]   K. K. Norton, J. Xu, and D. H. Gutmann, "Expression of the neurofibromatosis I gene product, neurofibromin, in blood vessel

endothelial cells and smooth muscle," *Neurobiol. Dis.*, vol. 2, no. 1, pp. 13–21, Feb. 1995.

[9]   B. Trovó-Marqui and E. H. Tajara, "Neurofibromin: a general outlook," *Clin. Genet.*, vol. 70, no. 1, pp. 1–13, Jul. 2006.

[10] E. Denayer, T. de Ravel, and E. Legius, "Clinical and molecular aspects of RAS related disorders," *J. Med. Genet.*, vol. 45, no. 11, pp. 695–703, Nov. 2008.

[11] J. Friedman, "Neurofibromatosis 1," in GeneReviews(®), R. A. Pagon, M. P. Adam, H. H. Ardinger, T. D. Bird, C. R. Dolan, C.-T. Fong, R. J. Smith, and K. Stephens, Eds. Seattle (WA): University of Washington, Seattle, 1993.

[12] K. N. Shah, "The diagnostic and clinical significance of café-au-lait macules," Pediatr. *Clin. North Am.*, vol. 57, no. 5, pp. 1131–1153, Oct. 2010.

[13] J. H. Tonsgard, "Clinical manifestations and management of neurofibromatosis type 1," *Semin. Pediatr. Neurol.*, vol. 13, no. 1, pp. 2–7, Mar. 2006.

[14] D. G. R. Evans, C. O'Hara, A. Wilding, S. L. Ingham, E. Howard, J. Dawson, A. Moran, V. Scott-Kitching, F. Holt, and S. M. Huson, "Mortality in neurofibromatosis 1: in North West England: an assessment of actuarial survival in a region of the UK since 1989," Eur. *J. Hum. Genet.*, vol. 19, no. 11, pp. 1187–1191, Nov. 2011.

[15] S. A. Rasmussen, Q. Yang, and J. M. Friedman, "Mortality in Neurofibromatosis 1: An Analysis Using U.S. Death Certificates," Am. *J. Hum. Genet.*, vol. 68, no. 5, pp. 1110–1118, May 2001.

[16] M. Zöller, B. Rembeck, H. O. Akesson, and L. Angervall, "Life expectancy, mortality and prognostic factors in neurofibromatosis type 1. A twelve-year follow-up of an epidemiological study in Göteborg, Sweden," *Acta Derm. Venereol.*, vol. 75, no. 2, pp. 136–140, Mar. 1995.

[17] G. S. Oderich, T. M. Sullivan, T. C. Bower, P. Gloviczki, D. V. Miller, D. Babovic-Vuksanovic, T. A. Macedo, and A. Stanson, "Vascular abnormalities in patients with neurofibromatosis syndrome type I: clinical spectrum, management, and results," *J. Vasc. Surg.*, vol. 46, no. 3, pp. 475–484, Sep. 2007.

[18] B. Kaas, T. A. G. M. Huisman, A. Tekes, A. Bergner, J. O. Blakeley, and L. C. Jordan, "Spectrum and prevalence of vasculopathy in pediatric neurofibromatosis type 1," *J. Child Neurol.*, vol. 28, no. 5, pp. 561–569, May 2013.

[19] M. Fujimoto, I. Nakahara, M. Tanaka, Y. Iwamuro, Y. Watanabe, and K. Harada, "[Multiple intracranial aneurysms and vascular abnormalities associated with neurofibromatosis type 1: a case report]," *No Shinkei Geka.*, vol. 32, no. 4, pp. 355–359, Apr. 2004.

[20] M. H. Gorelick, C. M. Powell, K. N. Rosenbaum, H. M. Saal, J. Conry, and C. R. Fitz, "Progressive occlusive cerebrovascular disease in a patient with neurofibromatosis type 1," *Clin. Pediatr.* (Phila.), vol. 31, no. 5, pp. 313–315, May 1992.

[21] P. Cluzel, L. Pierot, A. Leung, A. Gaston, E. Kieffer, and J. Chiras, "Vertebral arteriovenous fistulae in neurofibromatosis: report of two cases and review of the literature," *Neuroradiology*, vol. 36, no. 4, pp. 321–325, May 1994.

[22] J. K. Podgórski, B. Kalicki, S. Długoborska, J. Rafińska, A. Kadłubowski, A. Jung, and A. Koziarskiego, "[Difficulties in the diagnosis of cerebral abscess in a 15-year old boy with von Recklinghausen disease treated surgically: recovery case report]," *Neurol. Neurochir. Pol.,* vol. 29, no. 4, pp. 623–629, Aug. 1995.

[23] E. J. Piovesan, R. H. Scola, L. C. Werneck, V. H. Zétola, E. M. Nóvak, F. M. Iwamoto, and L. M. Piovesan, "Neurofibromatosis, stroke and basilar impression. Case report," *Arq. Neuropsiquiatr.*, vol. 57, no. 2B, pp. 484–488, Jun. 1999.

[24] E. Sareli and D. S. Marshall, "A Devastating Complication of Type 1 Neurofibromatosis," *Am. J. Respir. Crit. Care Med.*, vol. 185, no. 9, pp. e12–e13, May 2012.

[25] G. Rosenbusch, W. H. Hoefinagels, R. A. Koene, W. Penn, and H. O. Thijssen, "[Renovascular hypertension in neurofibromatosis. Simultaneous occurrence of multiple abdominal and cerebral vascular abnormalities (author's transl)]," *RöFo Fortschritte Auf Dem Geb. Röntgenstrahlen Nukl.*, vol. 126, no. 3, pp. 218–227, Mar. 1977.

[26] J. F. Rizzo 3rd and S. Lessell, "Cerebrovascular abnormalities in neurofibromatosis type 1," *Neurology,* vol. 44, no. 6, pp. 1000–1002, Jun. 1994.

[27] J. M. Friedman, J. Arbiser, J. A. Epstein, D. H. Gutmann, S. J. Huot, A. E. Lin, B. Mcmanus, and B. R. Korf, "Cardiovascular disease in neurofibromatosis 1: Report of the NF1 Cardiovascular Task Force," *Genet. Med.,* vol. 4, no. 3, pp. 105–111, May 2002.

[28] E. Lin, P. H. Birch, B. R. Korf, R. Tenconi, M. Niimura, M. Poyhonen, K. Armfield Uhas, M. Sigorini, R. Virdis, C. Romano, E. Bonioli, P. Wolkenstein, E. K. Pivnick, M. Lawrence, and J. M. Friedman,

"Cardiovascular malformations and other cardiovascular abnormalities in neurofibromatosis 1," *Am. J. Med. Genet.*, vol. 95, no. 2, pp. 108–117, Nov. 2000.

[29] Y. J. Park, K. M. Park, J. Oh, H. S. Park, J.-S. Kim, and Y.-W. Kim, "Spontaneous aortic rupture in a patient with neurofibromatosis type 1," *J. Korean Surg. Soc.*, vol. 82, no. 4, pp. 261–265, Apr. 2012.

[30] P. S. Ghosh, A. D. Rothner, T. M. Emch, N. R. Friedman, and M. Moodley, "Cerebral vasculopathy in children with neurofibromatosis type 1," *J. Child Neurol.*, vol. 28, no. 1, pp. 95–101, Jan. 2013.

[31] F. D'Arco, A. D'Amico, F. Caranci, N. D. Paolo, D. Melis, and A. Brunetti, "Cerebrovascular stenosis in neurofibromatosis type 1 and utility of magnetic resonance angiography: our experience and literature review," *Radiol. Med.* (Torino), vol. 119, no. 6, pp. 415–421, Jun. 2014.

[32] T. Lehrnbecher, A. M. Gassel, V. Rauh, T. Kirchner, and H. I. Huppertz, "Neurofibromatosis presenting as a severe systemic vasculopathy," *Eur. J. Pediatr.*, vol. 153, no. 2, pp. 107–109, Feb. 1994.

[33] J. F. Greene Jr, J. E. Fitzwater, and J. Burgess, "Arterial lesions associated with neurofibromatosis," *Am. J. Clin. Pathol.*, vol. 62, no. 4, pp. 481–487, Oct. 1974.

[34] M. Halpern and G. Currarino, "Vascular Lesions Causing Hypertension in Neurofibromatosis*,*" *N. Engl. J. Med.*, vol. 273, no. 5, pp. 248–252, 1965.

[35] F. Reubi, "Les vaisseaux et les glandes endocrines dans la neurofibromatose.," *Pathobiology,* vol. 7, no. 3, pp. 168–236, 1944.

[36] M. G. Muhonen, J. C. Godersky, and J. C. VanGilder, "Cerebral aneurysms associated with neurofibromatosis," *Surg. Neurol.*, vol. 36, no. 6, pp. 470–475, Dec. 1991.

[37] J. Z. Zhao and X. D. Han, "Cerebral aneurysm associated with von Recklinghausen's neurofibromatosis: a case report," *Surg. Neurol.*, vol. 50, no. 6, pp. 592–596, Dec. 1998.

[38] B. L. Smith, C. E. Munschauer, N. Diamond, and F. Rivera, "Ruptured internal carotid aneurysm resulting from neurofibromatosis: treatment with intraluminal stent graft," *J. Vasc. Surg.*, vol. 32, no. 4, pp. 824–828, Oct. 2000.

[39] J. A. Ahlgren-Beckendorf, W. W. Maggio, F. Chen, and T. A. Kent, "Neurofibromatosis 1 mRNA expression in blood vessels," *Biochem. Biophys. Res. Commun.*, vol. 197, no. 2, pp. 1019–1024, Dec. 1993.

[40] T. L. Rosser, G. Vezina, and R. J. Packer, "Cerebrovascular abnormalities in a population of children with neurofibromatosis type 1," *Neurology*, vol. 64, no. 3, pp. 553–555, Feb. 2005.

[41] J. E. Deanfield, J. P. Halcox, and T. J. Rabelink, "Endothelial Function and Dysfunction Testing and Clinical Relevance," *Circulation*, vol. 115, no. 10, pp. 1285–1295, Mar. 2007.

[42] V. M. Riccardi, "Histogenesis control genes and neurofibromatosis 1," *Eur. J. Pediatr.*, vol. 159, no. 7, pp. 475–476, Jul. 2000.

[43] J. Xu, F. A. Ismat, T. Wang, J. Yang, and J. A. Epstein, "NF1 regulates a Ras-dependent vascular smooth muscle proliferative injury response," *Circulation,* vol. 116, no. 19, pp. 2148–2156, Nov. 2007.

[44] G. Cairns and K. N. North, "Cerebrovascular dysplasia in neurofibromatosis type 1," *J. Neurol. Neurosurg. Psychiatry*, vol. 79, no. 10, pp. 1165–1170, Oct. 2008.

[45] R. M. Scott and E. R. Smith, "Moyamoya Disease and Moyamoya Syndrome," *N. Engl. J. Med.*, vol. 360, no. 12, pp. 1226–1237, 2009.

[46] E. R. Smith and R. M. Scott, "Moyamoya: epidemiology, presentation, and diagnosis," Neurosurg. *Clin. N. Am.*, vol. 21, no. 3, pp. 543–551, Jul. 2010.

[47] Duat-Rodríguez, F. Carceller Lechón, M. Á. López Pino, C. Rodríguez Fernández, and L. González-Gutiérrez-Solana, "Neurofibromatosis type 1 associated with moyamoya syndrome in children," *Pediatr. Neurol.*, vol. 50, no. 1, pp. 96–98, Jan. 2014.

[48] M. Koss, R. M. Scott, M. B. Irons, E. R. Smith, and N. J. Ullrich, "Moyamoya syndrome associated with neurofibromatosis Type 1: perioperative and long-term outcome after surgical revascularization," *J. Neurosurg. Pediatr.*, vol. 11, no. 4, pp. 417–425, Feb. 2013.

[49] D. Rea, J. F. Brandsema, D. Armstrong, P. C. Parkin, G. deVeber, D. MacGregor, W. J. Logan, and R. Askalan, "Cerebral arteriopathy in children with neurofibromatosis type 1," *Pediatrics,* vol. 124, no. 3, pp. e476–483, Sep. 2009.

[50] T. Yamauchi, M. Tada, K. Houkin, T. Tanaka, Y. Nakamura, S. Kuroda, H. Abe, T. Inoue, K. Ikezaki, T. Matsushima, and M. Fukui, "Linkage of familial moyamoya disease (spontaneous occlusion of the circle of Willis) to chromosome 17q25," *Stroke J. Cereb. Circ.*, vol. 31, no. 4, pp. 930–935, Apr. 2000.

[51] B. R. Korf, "Malignancy in Neurofibromatosis Type 1," The Oncologist, vol. 5, no. 6, pp. 477–485, Dec. 2000.

[52] N. J. Ullrich, M. Zimmerman, E. Smith, M. Irons, K. Marcus, and M. W. Kieran, "Association of rapidly progressive moyamoya syndrome with bevacizumab treatment for glioblastoma in a child with neurofibromatosis type 1," *J. Child Neurol.,* vol. 26, no. 2, pp. 228–230, Feb. 2011.

[53] W. I. Schievink, M. Riedinger, and M. M. Maya, "Frequency of incidental intracranial aneurysms in neurofibromatosis type 1," *Am. J. Med. Genet.* A., vol. 134A, no. 1, pp. 45–48, Apr. 2005.

[54] M. W. You, E. J. Kim, and W. S. Choi, "Intracranial and extracranial fusiform aneurysms in a patient with neurofibromatosis type 1: a case report," *Neurointervention,* vol. 6, no. 1, pp. 34–37, Feb. 2011.

[55] J. Baldauf, J. Kiwit, and M. Synowitz, "Cerebral aneurysms associated with von Recklinghausen's neurofibromatosis: report of a case and review of the literature," Neurol. India, vol. 53, no. 2, pp. 213–215, Jun. 2005.

[56] G. Lassmann, "Vascular dysplasia of arteries in neurocristopathies: a lesson for neurofibromatosis," *Neurofibromatosis,* vol. 1, no. 5–6, pp. 281–293, 1988.

[57] J. L. Fox, Intracranial aneurysms. Springer-Verlag, 1983.

[58] E. Sobata, H. Ohkuma, and S. Suzuki, "Cerebrovascular disorders associated with von Recklinghausen's neurofibromatosis: a case report," Neurosurgery, vol. 22, no. 3, pp. 544–549, Mar. 1988.

[59] M. Salcman, E. Botero, and E. Bellis, "Giant posttraumatic aneurysm of the intracranial carotid artery: evolution and regression documented by computed tomography," *Neurosurgery*, vol. 16, no. 2, pp. 218–221, Feb. 1985.

[60] T. Kubota, H. Nakai, T. Tanaka, T. Maeda, K. Takano, N. Tsuda, N. Izumi, N. Ogata, and K. Goto, "A case of intracranial arteriovenous fistula in an infant with neurofibromatosis type 1," Childs Nerv. Syst. ChNS Off. *J. Int. Soc. Pediatr. Neurosurg.*, vol. 18, no. 3–4, pp. 166–170, Apr. 2002.

[61] J. E. Cohen, J. M. Gomori, S. Grigoriadis, S. Spektor, and G. Rajz, "Dural arteriovenous fistula of the greater sphenoid wing region in neurofibromatosis type 1," *Pediatr. Neurosurg.*, vol. 44, no. 2, pp. 172–175, 2008.

[62] G. Higa, J. P. Pacanowski Jr, D. T. Jeck, K. R. Goshima, and L. R. León Jr, "Vertebral artery aneurysms and cervical arteriovenous fistulae in patients with neurofibromatosis 1," *Vascular*, vol. 18, no. 3, pp. 166–177, Jun. 2010.

[63] H. M. Liu, H. C. Shih, Y. C. Huang, and Y. H. Wang, "Posterior cranial fossa arteriovenous fistula with presenting as caroticocavernous fistula," *Neuroradiology*, vol. 43, no. 5, pp. 405–408, May 2001.

[64] W. R. Deans, S. Bloch, L. Leibrock, B. M. Berman, and F. M. Skultety, "Arteriovenous fistula in patients with neurofibromatosis," *Radiology*, vol. 144, no. 1, pp. 103–107, Jul. 1982.

[65] L. Lin and D. H. Gutmann, "Advances in the treatment of neurofibromatosis-associated tumours," *Nat. Rev. Clin. Oncol.*, vol. 10, no. 11, pp. 616–624, Nov. 2013.

[66] V. Leier, C. J. Dewan, and L. F. Anatasia, "Fatal Hemorrhage as a Complication of Neurofibromatosis," *Vasc. Endovascular Surg.*, vol. 6, no. 2, pp. 98–101, Mar. 1972.

[67] Nopajaroonsri and A. A. Lurie, "Venous aneurysm, arterial dysplasia, and near-fatal hemorrhages in neurofibromatosis type 1," *Hum. Pathol.*, vol. 27, no. 9, pp. 982–985, Sep. 1996.

[68] V. Kumar, Robbins & Cotran Pathologic Basis of Disease: With STUDENT CONSULT Online Access, 8e, 8th edition. Philadelphia, PA: Saunders, 2009.

[69] K. A. Robertson, G. Nalepa, F.-C. Yang, D. C. Bowers, C. Y. Ho, G. D. Hutchins, J. M. Croop, T. A. Vik, S. C. Denne, L. F. Parada, C. M. Hingtgen, L. E. Walsh, M. Yu, K. R. Pradhan, M. K. Edwards-Brown, M. D. Cohen, J. W. Fletcher, J. B. Travers, K. W. Staser, M. W. Lee, M. R. Sherman, C. J. Davis, L. C. Miller, D. A. Ingram, and D. W. Clapp, "Imatinib mesylate for plexiform neurofibromas in patients with neurofibromatosis type 1: a phase 2 trial," *Lancet Oncol.*, vol. 13, no. 12, pp. 1218–1224, Dec. 2012.

In: Neurofibromatosis ISBN: 978-1-63463-229-4
Editor: Walter Romaine © 2015 Nova Science Publishers, Inc.

Chapter 4

TARGETING THE TUMOR MICROENVIRONMENT FOR THE TREATMENT OF PLEXIFORM NEUROFIBROMAS IN PATIENTS WITH NEUROFIBROMATOSIS TYPE 1

Mia Yang Chen, Steven David Rhodes and David Wade Clapp

Herman B Wells Center for Pediatric Research, Departments of Pediatrics,
Indiana University School of Medicine, Indianapolis, Indiana, US

ABSTRACT

Neurofibromatosis type 1 (NF1) affects 1 in 3,500 people and is one of the most common genetic disorders with a predisposition to malignancy. NF1 is caused by autosomal dominant mutations in the *NF1* tumor suppressor gene, which encodes neurofibromin, a negative regulator of Ras-activity. Cutaneous and plexiform neurofibromas, the hallmark tumors of NF1, are heterogeneous neoplasms composed of tumorigenic Schwann cells and a complex microenvironment, including mast cells, fibroblasts, and blood vessels. Emerging evidence indicates a pivotal role for interactions between Schwann cells, surrounding stroma, and hematopoietic constituents of the tumor microenvironment in promoting neurofibroma genesis. In NF1 mouse models, tumorigenic *Nf1* nullizygous Schwan cells secrete supraphysiologic levels of stem cell factor (SCF), co-opting *Nf1* haploinsufficient mast cells to infiltrate the tumor microenvironment. In turn, activated $Nf1^{+/-}$ mast cells secrete multiple inflammatory effectors which potentiate fibroblast proliferation, collagen deposition and angiogenesis, thereby creating a viscous cycle perpetuating neurofibroma maintenance and expansion. Experimental evidence from NF1 murine models indicates that either genetic or pharmacologic inhibition of SCF/c-kit dependent mast cell recruitment/activation is sufficient to treat neurofibromas in the NF1 murine model. A recent phase 2 clinical trial using Gleevec, which targets multi-tyrosine kinases including c-kit, provided the first evidence of an effective therapy for the treatment of plexiform neurofibromas. This chapter will review current clinical and animal model data delineating the role of the tumor microenvironment in neurofibroma pathogenesis and therapy.

1. TUMOR MICROENVIRONMENTS

It has been established that chronic inflammation increases susceptibility to many forms of cancer, a concept first proposed in 1863 by Rudolf Virchow when he postulated sites of chronic inflammation to be a putative source of origin for cancer [1]. Virchow's idea stemmed from his observations that certain classes of irritants in combination with tissue injury enhanced cell proliferation [2]. While cancer stem cells within the tumor carry the oncogenic and tumor suppressor mutations that define cancer as a genetic disease, the tumor is also composed of multiple cell types, including fibroblasts, immune cells (such as mast cells), endothelial cells, and blood vessels among other lineages which comprise the tumor microenvironment [1, 3]. Experimental evidence has since confirmed the tumor microenvironment to be an integral component of the neoplastic process, perpetuating cellular proliferation, survival, and metastasis [3].

Critical to the formation of tumor-associated vasculature, endothelial cells are a central constituent of the tumor microenvironment [3]. Activated by the "angionenic switch", quiescent endothelial cells are reprogramed to generate new blood vessels, providing nutrients and oxygen to the growing tumor. VEGF, angiopietin, FGF, and Notch pathways [4, 5] are among the more well-known signaling effectors that have been implicated the co-option of endothelial cells within the tumor microenvironment – a subject which remains an area of active investigation.

Pericytes are a specialized mesenchymal cell population within the tumor microenvironment which interface with tumor-associated vasculature by producing cytoplasmic projections that engulf and provide paracrine support signals to endothelial cells [3, 6, 7]. Together with endothelial cells, they provide an anchoring vascular basement membrane which reinforces blood vessel walls against the hydrostatic forces of blood flow [3]. Recent genetic and pharmacologic data demonstrate that disruption of pericyte recruitment and function destabilizes vascular integrity, thereby enabling cancer cells to gain access to tumor-associated vasculature and promoting hematogenous metastasis [3, 7-10].

Fibroblasts are one of the predominant cell populations within cancer microenvironments and can be further subcategorized into two subtypes: cells similar to fibroblasts that provide foundational support to normal epithelial tissues and myofibroblasts, which express α-smooth muscle actin (SMA) are present in increasing numbers within sites of chronic inflammation [3]. While myofibroblasts are beneficial to tissue repair, they can have deleterious effects in chronic inflammation, leading to pathological fibrosis in certain tissues. In addition, recruited myofibroblasts have been implicated in perpetuating multiple neoplastic processes including proliferation, angiogenesis, invasion, and metastasis [11-14].

Inflammatory cells of the immune system have become increasing recognized as a pivotal component of the tumor microenvironment. Such cell types include neutrophils, and lymphocytes, macrophages, and mast cells. Expressing a diverse array of cytokines including EGF, VEGF, and FGF as well as other effector molecules including matrix metaloproteinases (MMPs) which have been demonstrated to facilitate angiogenesis, stimulate proliferation, and promote tumor invasion and metastasis among other functions [3, 15-20]. This chapter will review emerging evidence demonstrating that infiltrating inflammatory cells within the tumor microenvironment pivotally underpin plexiform neurofibroma pathogenesis.

2. NF1 GENETICS AND MANIFESTATIONS

NF1, also known as von Recklinghausen's disease, is caused by mutations in the *NF1* tumor suppressor gene located on chromosome 17q11.2 [21, 22]. Spanning over 350 kb of genomic DNA and containing at least 60 exons [23], NF1 encodes the protein neurofibromin which functions as a GTPase activating protein (GAP) for Ras, accelerating the hydrolysis of Ras from its active GTP- to inactive GDP-bound conformation [21, 24]. NF1 affects approximately 1 in 3,500 individuals worldwide and is also the most common genetic disorder with a predisposition to cancer [25]. *NF1* mutations are inherited in an autosomal dominant fashion although spontaneous mutations are believed to account for approximately 50 percent of cases [26]. Although NF1 has traditionally been characterized as a disorder of neural-crest derived tissues (Schwann cells, glia, melanocytes, etc.), the disorder is now recognized to give rise to a wide spectrum of malignant and non-malignant clinical presentations arising from all embryonic germ layers. These manifestations include café au lait macules (areas of skin hyperpigmentation), Lisch nodules (hamartomas on the iris), axillary and groin freckling, peripheral and central nerve tumors, myeloid leukemia, pheochromocytomas, learning deficits, vasculopathies, and skeletal anomalies [25][27]. Thus, NF1 can be characterized as both a syndrome with a predisposition to cancer as well as a disease affecting systemic development.

Neurofibromas are the hallmark tumor of NF1 and can be subclassified into distinct subtypes based on their anatomical compartmentalization. Cutaneous and subcutaneous neurofibromas occur nearly universally in all NF1 patients and arise from peripheral nerve fibers during adolescence. Although typically benign, disfigurement which often occurs as the burden of dermal neurofibromas continues to increase with age can lead to significant morbidity. By contrast, plexiform neurofibromas are congenital and occur with approximately 30 percent penetrance [28], arising from the cranial and large peripheral nerve sheaths. As these tumors continue to enlarge, they lead to significant morbidity and mortality by compressing the cranial and/or paraspinal peripheral nerve roots. Associated symptoms include paresthesias, paralysis, respiratory compromise, as well as bowel and bladder dysfunction [29, 30]. Plexiform neurofibromas are also associated with a 10 percent lifetime incidence of transformation to malignant peripheral nerve sheath tumors (MPNSTs) which can lead rapidly to death through widespread metastasis [31, 32].

Neurofibromas are heterogeneous tumors comprised of Schwann cells, fibroblasts, vascular cells and infiltrating mast cells [33-37]. Mast cells are immune effector cells derived from common myeloid progenitor cells of the hematopoietic system [38]. Stem cell factor (SCF) signaling through its receptor tyrosine kinase c-kit has been demonstrated to be an indispensable requirement for mast cell cytopoiesis, whereby *W* (white spotting locus mice) harboring naturally acquired *c-kit* mutations are profoundly mast cell deficient [39-41]. Aside from their canonical immunomodulatory functions in allergy and asthma, the pro-inflammatory effects of activated mast cells have been demonstrated to play a significant role within tumor microenvironments, perpetuating multiple neoplastic processes including extracellular matrix remodeling, tumor growth, invasion, and metastasis [1, 42, 43]. While mast cells have been widely recognized as a hallmark histological feature of the neurofibroma since the 1980s, their functional significance with respect to neurofibroma initiation and maintenance has only recently been realized.

The concept that mast cells may pivotally underpin neurofibroma genesis was first postulated by Vincent Riccardi, based on his clinical observations of concomitant pruritus associated with dermal neurofibromas [44]. Consistent with these findings, early clinical trials testing ketotifen, a mast cell granule stabilizer, demonstrated anti-puritic effects but did not appear to curb neurofibroma growth [45, 46] – suggesting that inhibition of mast cell degranulation alone is insufficient to impact disease progression. The remainder of this chapter will discuss recent experimental evidence from mouse and human studies demonstrating a critical role for SCF/c-kit dependent mast cell gain in-functions in engendering neurofibroma growth and progression.

3. MODELING NEUROFIBROMAS IN THE MOUSE

Studies utilizing transgenic NF1 mouse models have dramatically enhanced our understanding of the contribution of the tumor microenvironment to neurofibroma genesis. Mice nullizygous for *Nf1* die prior to embryonic day 13.5 secondary to cardiac outflow tract anomalies but do exhibit hyperplasia of neural crest-derived sympathetic ganglia [47]. By contrast, *Nf1* heterozygoous mice (*Nf1*$^{+/-}$) are viable into adulthood but do exhibit an increased predisposition malignancies including pheochromocytomas and myeloid leukemia after approximately 1 year of life secondary to loss of heterozygosity (LOH) of the WT *Nf1* allele in affected tissue [48]. Intriguingly however, these animals do not develop hallmark dermal or plexiform neurofibromas characteristic of the human disease. One plausible explanation for this fundamental discrepancy relates to the shortened timespan window for LOH to initiate neurofibroma genesis in the necessary tumorigenic cells of origin during the murine gestation and lifecycle.

The requirement for *Nf1* LOH as a prerequisite for neurofibroma formation was first demonstrated by Cichowski and colleagues whereby chimeric mice were generated by injection of *Nf1*$^{-/-}$ embryonic stem cells into WT blastocysts [49]. These *Nf1*$^{-/-}$ chimeric mice exhibited neurofibromas at multiple nerve levels recapitulating many of the characteristic histopathological features of human neurofibromas. While these studies solidified the requirement of *Nf1* homozygosity for neurofibroma formation and affirmed the role of *Nf1* as a tumor suppressor, delineation of a tumor cell of origin remained infeasible by this approach. In addition, the *Nf1*$^{-/-}$ chimera model does not accurately recapitulate the genetic status of human NF1 patients, where *NF1*$^{-/-}$ tumorigenic cells interact with a *NF1*$^{+/-}$ microenvironment. Thus, unanswered questions remained regarding the potential contribution of *NF1* gene dose in surrounding fibroblasts, pericytes, endothelial cells, and hematopoietic cells in neurofibroma pathogenesis.

The embryonic lethality of germline *Nf1* nullizygosity and the inherent limitations of the *Nf1*$^{-/-}$ chimera model prompted Zhu and colleagues to adopt a more elegant approach utilizing Cre/loxP technology to allow tissue specific *Nf1* genetic ablation [50]. In this system, loxP sites flanking *Nf1* exon 31 and 32 were inserted, permitting Cre-mediated recombination of *Nf1* in a lineage restricted fashion. Genetic intercross of *Nf1*$^{flox/flox}$ mice with transgenic animals expressing Cre under the *Krox20*, embryonic Schwann cell specific promoter generated mutants harboring conditional *Nf1* nullizygosity in Schwann cells, the purported neurofibroma tumor cell of origin. Puzzlingly, *Nf1*$^{flox/flox}$;*Krox20Cre* mice failed to develop pathognomonic neurofibromas observed in the human disease, suggesting that Schwann cell *Nf1* LOH alone is insufficient for neurofibroma genesis, but rather, haploinsufficiency of *Nf1* within the tumor microenvironment may also be required to engender neurofibroma development.

4. MICROENVIRONMENT INTERACTIONS PERPETUATE NEUROFIBROMA PROGRESSION

Indeed, when *Nf1*$^{flox/flox}$;*Krox20Cre* mice were intercrossed with germline *Nf1*$^{+/-}$ mice to generate *Nf1*$^{flox/-}$;*Krox20Cre* animals harboring *Nf1* nullizygous Schwann cells on a *Nf1*$^{+/-}$ background, these animals develop diffuse enlargement of peripheral nerve roots along the dorsal spinal column closely reminiscent of human plexiform neurofibroma tissue both morphologically and histopathologically – featuring dysplastic Schwann cells, fibroblast proliferation, collagen deposition, and an abundance of infiltrating mast cells [50]. These genetic data confirmed *Nf1* nullizygous Schwann cells as the tumor cell of origin required for neurofibroma genesis while demonstrating a critical role for *Nf1* haploinsufficiency within the tumor microenvironment in perpetuating neurofibroma development.

The observation of infiltrating mast cells as a predominant histopathological feature of plexiform neurofibromas coupled with genetic evidence that neurofibroma development and progression in murine models requires cooperative interactions between $Nf1^{-/-}$ Schwann cells and an *Nf1* haploinsufficient microenvironment implicated *Nf1* heterozygous mast cells as critical mediators in neurofibroma genesis. Yet the mechanisms by which $Nf1^{+/-}$ mast cells are recruited to the neurofibroma microenvironment and function to perpetuate tumor development remained unclear. In 2003, Yang et al. demonstrated that $Nf1^{-/-}$ Schwann cells secrete 6-fold increased levels of stem cell factor (SCF), a potent chemoattractant for recruitment of bone marrow derived mast cells to the neurofibroma microenvironment [51]. *Nf1* haploinsufficient ($Nf1^{+/-}$) mast cells, in turn, exhibit increased chemotaxis [51] and degranulation [52] in response to SCF-dependent c-kit signaling, mediated by hyperactivation of the Ras-Raf-Mek-Erk and PI3K-Rac-Pak1-p38 [53] signaling axes. Experimental evidence also indicates that hyperactive p21-Ras-PI3K signaling confers resistance to apoptosis by suppressing Fas antigen expression in SCF stimulated mast cells [54], thereby potentiating $Nf1^{+/-}$ mast cell survival.

Upon entering the tumor microenvironment, SCF stimulated $Nf1^{+/-}$ mast cells function to perpetuate tumorigenesis in a paracrine fashion by hypersecreting a number of mitogenic substances. One such cytokine, transforming growth factor-beta (TGF-β) is known to be a potent stimulus for fibroblast proliferation, migration and collagen synthesis. Fibroblasts represent a major cellular constituent of the neurofibroma microenvironment with their secreted collagen comprising nearly one-half the tumor dry weight [55]. Yang et al. demonstrated that $Nf1^{+/-}$ mast cells secrete supraphysiological levels of TGF-β, enhancing $Nf1^{+/-}$ fibroblast bioactivity and collagen deposition through Ras-dependent hyperactivation of c-abl kinase [56]. Additionally, mast cells are known to produce a number of angionenic factors including vascular endothelial growth factor (VEGF) and platelet derived growth factor BB (PDGF-BB) which have been postulated to facilitate a microenvironment permissive for tumorigenesis by promoting neovascularization. Consistent with this hypothesis, $Nf1^{+/-}$ endothelial cells [57] and vascular smooth muscle cells [58] have been demonstrated to exhibit increased migratory and proliferative responses to VEGF and PDGF-BB, respectively, mediated by Ras-dependent hyperactivation of the Raf-Mek-Erk pathway.

5. SCF/C-KIT ACTIVATED $Nf1^{+/-}$ MAST CELLS PIVOTALLY UNDERPIN PLEXIFORM NEURIBROMA GENESIS

Collectively, these experimental data provided the basis for a working model by which $Nf1$-deficient Schwann cells and infiltrating $Nf1$ haploinsufficient mast cells work together to co-opt other $Nf1^{+/-}$ cellular constituents within the neurofibroma microenvironment to promote tumorigenesis. Nonetheless, key questions remain regarding which specific $Nf1$ haploinsufficient cell types (mast cells, fibroblasts, endothelial cells, etc.) are required to engender neurofibroma formation. Through an elegant series of adoptive bone marrow transfer studies, Yang et al. addressed this question by transplanting $Nf1^{+/-}$ hematopoietic stem cells into lethally irradiated $Nf1^{flox/flox}$;Krox20Cre recipient mice (which physiologically do not develop neurofibromas) [59]. Intriguingly, after approximately 6 months of stable hematopoietic reconstitution, $Nf1^{flox/flox}$;Krox20Cre mice transplanted with $Nf1^{+/-}$ bone marrow cells developed diffuse enlargements along their dorsal root ganglia histopathologically reminiscent of human plexiform neurofibromas. Conversely, a rescue experiment was performed whereby transplantation of WT hematopoietic cells to lethally irradiated $Nf1^{flox/-}$;Krox20Cre mice prevented neurofibroma development in these animals [59]. Taken together, these data demonstrate that $Nf1$ haploinsufficiency within the hematopoietic compartment, in conjunction with $Nf1$ nullizygous Schwann cells, is both necessary and sufficient to induce plexiform neurofibromas.

To further delineate $Nf1^{+/-}$ SCF-stimulated mast cells as the principal hematopoietic effectors required to initiate neurofibroma genesis, additional transplantation studies were performed with bone marrow from mice harboring 2 different c-kit genetic mutations (W^v/W^v or W^{41}/W^{41}) resulting in profoundly deficient mast cell cytopoiesis [41, 60-62]. $Nf1^{flox/-}$;Krox20Cre mice reconstituted with c-kit mutant $Nf1^{+/-}$;W^v/W^v or $Nf1^{+/-}$;W^{41}/W^{41} hematopoietic cells did not develop neurofibromas. An engraftment efficiency of greater than 95% was confirmed by Southern blot analysis of genomic DNA isolated from myeloid colonies cultured from the bone marrow of recipient mice [59]. These data indicate plexiform neurofibroma genesis, in the context of Schwann cell $Nf1$ LOH, requires c-kit dependent $Nf1$ haploinsufficiency in the bone marrow, thus implicating $Nf1^{+/-}$ mast cells as the culprit hematopoietic mediators underpinning neurofibroma development.

6. PHARMACOLOGIC SCF/C-KIT INHIBITION IN THE TREATMENT OF PLEXIFORM NEUROFIBROMAS

In light of evidence implicating SCF-dependent c-kit signaling within *Nf1* haploinsufficient mast cells as a pivotal effector axis mediating plexiform neurofibroma genesis, Yang et al. proceeded to test whether pharmacologic c-kit inhibition could prevent neurofibroma growth and progression in the NF1 murine model. Imatinib mesylate, marketed under the trade name Gleevec, is a pharmacologic inhibitor of multiple tyrosine kinases including c-kit, PDGF-β, and bcr/abl and currently carries FDA approval for the treatment of Philadelphia chromosome positive chronic myelogenous leukemia (CML) and gastrointestinal stromal tumor (GIST) among other indications. Administration of imatinib mesylate to a cohort of *Nf1$^{flox/-}$;Krox20Cre* mice with pre-existing neurofibromas resulted in significant reductions in tumor volume and metabolic activity after three-months treatment. Histologically, dorsal root ganglia revealed decreased mast cell infiltration, a more organized Schwann cell architecture, enhanced apoptosis, and reduced proliferation as compared to placebo treated controls [59].

As the murine studies were nearing completion, a three year-old female with NF1 presented with life threatening airway compression resulting from a progressively enlarging plexiform neurofibroma involving the left floor of the oral cavity, neck, and mastoid bone with encasement of the carotid artery and jugular vein precluding surgical resection. Due to impending respiratory compromise and lack of alternative treatment options, therapy with imatinib mesylate was initiated under a compassionate use protocol after discussing the potential risks and benefits and obtaining informed consent from the patient's family. Serial MRI scans obtained prior to and following three-months treatment with 350 mg/m^2 imatinib mesylate revealed a reduction in tumor volume of approximately 70 percent with no adverse side effects. Significant symptomatic improvement with respect to the patient's drooling, insomnia, and anorexia were also noted [59].

This dramatic result, albeit from a single patient, in the context of analogous results demonstrated in the NF1 murine model, provided impetus for initiation of an open label phase 2 trial of imatinib mesylate for the treatment of plexiform neurofibromas in NF1. This study, directed by Robertson and colleagues enrolled 36 eligible patients aged 3-65 years with clinically significant plexiform neurofibromas on an intention to treat basis for a minimum duration of 6 months. Pediatric patients received oral imatinib at a dose of 220 mg/m^2 twice daily while adults received a 400 mg/m^2 twice daily dose. A 20 percent or greater reduction in tumor size, as determined by sequential volumetric MRI, was defined as the objective response threshold and primary endpoint. Of the 23 patients receiving imatinib for a minimum duration of 6 months, a reduction in tumor volume of at least 20 percent was observed in six of 23 patients [63]. Additional patients not meeting the objective response threshold were noted to have significant subjective and/or clinical improvement in their symptoms including improved airway patency, bladder control, and regain of neurological function [63]. Common adverse events included skin rash and oedema, with more serious side effects, such as reversible neutropenia, hyperglycemia and transaminitis occurring in a small subset of patients. Despite inherent limitations, the results of this study provide the first evidence of an effective therapy for the treatment of plexiform neurofibromas, validating previously published findings in the NF1 mouse model. Multicenter phase 3 trials are needed to validate the efficacy of imatinib mesylate in a larger NF1 patient population.

CONCLUSION

With the ability to accurately model hallmark NF1 disease manifestations in the mouse, our understanding of neurofibroma pathogenesis has increased dramatically over recent years. While many unanswered questions remain, deciphering the paracrine cross-talk networks by which $Nf1^{+/-}$ mast cells and other heterotypic cellular constituents of the microenvironment cooperate to induce neurofibroma formation has already begun to create opportunities for novel therapies. Here we have reviewed evidence that SCF/c-kit dependent mast cell activation pivotally underpins neurofibroma maintenance and progression by fostering an inflammatory microenvironment permissive for tumorigenesis. As insights gleaned from increasing sophisticated animal models of the disease continue to inform our mechanistic understanding of neurofibroma biology, our ability to medically manage the tremendous morbidity associated with these tumors will undoubtedly continue to improve.

Targeting the Tumor Microenvironment for the Treatment ...   75

REFERENCES

[1]   Coussens, LM; Werb, Z. Inflammation and cancer. *Nature*, 2002, 420(6917) 860-7,

[2]   Balkwill, F; Mantovani, A. Inflammation and cancer: back to Virchow? *Lancet*, 2001, 357(9255), 539-45,

[3]   Hanahan, D; Weinberg, RA. Hallmarks of cancer: the next generation. *Cell*, 2011, 144(5), 646-74,

[4]   Ahmed, Z; Bicknell, R. Angiogenic signalling pathways. *Methods Mol Biol*, 2009, 467, 3-24,

[5]   Carmeliet, P; Jain, RK. Angiogenesis in cancer and other diseases. *Nature*, 2000, 407(6801), 249-57,

[6]   Bergers, G; Song, S. The role of pericytes in blood-vessel formation and maintenance. *Neuro Oncol*, 2005, 7(4), 452-64,

[7]   Gaengel, K; et al., Endothelial-mural cell signaling in vascular development and angiogenesis. *Arterioscler Thromb Vasc Biol*, 2009, 29(5), 630-8,

[8]   Gerhardt, H; Semb, H. Pericytes: gatekeepers in tumour cell metastasis? *J Mol Med (Berl)*, 2008, 86(2), 135-44,

[9]   Pietras, K; Ostman, A. Hallmarks of cancer: interactions with the tumor stroma. *Exp Cell Res*, 2010, 316(8), 1324-31,

[10] Raza, A; Franklin, MJ; Dudek, AZ. Pericytes and vessel maturation during tumor angiogenesis and metastasis. *Am J Hematol*, 2010, 85(8), 593-8,

[11] Bhowmick, NA; Neilson, EG; Moses, HL. Stromal fibroblasts in cancer initiation and progression. *Nature*, 2004, 432(7015), 332-7,

[12] Kalluri, R; Zeisberg, M. Fibroblasts in cancer. *Nat Rev Cancer*, 2006, 6(5), 392-401,

[13] Rasanen, K; Vaheri, A. Activation of fibroblasts in cancer stroma. *Exp Cell Res*, 2010, 316(17), 2713-22,

[14] Shimoda, M; Mellody, KT; Orimo, A. Carcinoma-associated fibroblasts are a rate-limiting determinant for tumour progression. *Semin Cell Dev Biol*, 2010, 21(1), 19-25,

[15] Coffelt, SB; et al., Elusive identities and overlapping phenotypes of proangiogenic myeloid cells in tumors. *Am J Pathol*, 2010, 176(4), 1564-76,

[16] Joyce, JA; Pollard, JW. Microenvironmental regulation of metastasis. *Nat Rev Cancer*, 2009, 9(4), 239-52,

[17] Mantovani, A. Molecular pathways linking inflammation and cancer. *Curr Mol Med*, 2010, 10(4), 369-73,

[18] Mantovani, A; et al., Cancer-related inflammation. *Nature*, 2008, 454(7203), 436-44,

[19] Murdoch, C; et al., The role of myeloid cells in the promotion of tumour angiogenesis. *Nat Rev Cancer*, 2008, 8(8), 618-31,

[20] Qian, BZ; Pollard, JW. Macrophage diversity enhances tumor progression and metastasis. *Cell*, 2010, 141(1), 39-51,

[21] Ballester, R; et al., The NF1 locus encodes a protein functionally related to mammalian GAP and yeast IRA proteins. *Cell*, 1990, 63(4), 851-9,

[22] Xu, GF; et al., The neurofibromatosis type 1 gene encodes a protein related to GAP. *Cell*, 1990, 62(3), 599-608,

[23] Jentarra, G; Snyder, SL; Narayanan, V. Genetic aspects of neurocutaneous disorders. *Semin Pediatr Neurol*, 2006, 13(1), 43-7,

[24] Martin, GA., et al., The GAP-related domain of the neurofibromatosis type 1 gene product interacts with ras p21, Cell, 1990, 63(4), 843-9,

[25] Friedman, J; et al., Neurofibromatosis: phenotype, natural history, and pathogenesis. 3rd ed. Baltimore, MD: The Johns Hopkins University Press, 1999,

[26] Yohay, KH. The genetic and molecular pathogenesis of NF1 and NF2, *Semin Pediatr Neurol*, 2006, 13(1), 21-6,

[27] Bader, JL. Neurofibromatosis and cancer. *Ann N Y Acad Sci*, 1986, 486: 57-65,

[28] Le, LQ; Parada, LF. Tumor microenvironment and neurofibromatosis type I: connecting the GAPs. *Oncogene*, 2007, 26(32), 4609-16,

[29] Raffensperger, J; Cohen, R. Plexiform neurofibromas in childhood. *J Pediatr Surg*, 1972, 7(2), 144-51,

[30] Serletis, D; et al., Massive plexiform neurofibromas in childhood: natural history and management issues. *J Neurosurg*, 2007, 106(5 Suppl), 363-7,

[31] Ferner, RE. Neurofibromatosis 1, *Eur J Hum Genet*, 2007, 15(2), 131-8,

[32] Lakkis, MM; Tennekoon, GI. Neurofibromatosis type 1, I. General overview. *J Neurosci Res*, 2000, 62(6), 755-63,

[33] Baroni, C. On the Relationship of Mast Cells to Various Soft Tissue Tumours. *Br J Cancer*, 1964, 18: 686-91,

[34] Gamble, HJ; Goldby, S. Mast cells in peripheral nerve trunks. *Nature*, 1961, 189: 766-7,

[35] Isaacson, P. Mast cells in benign nerve sheath tumours. *J Pathol*, 1976, 119(4), 193-6,

[36] Olsson, Y. Mast cells in human peripheral nerve. *Acta Neurol Scand*, 1971, 47(3), 357-68,

[37] Pineda, A. Mast cells--their presence and ultrastructural characteristics in peripheral nerve tumors. *Arch Neurol*, 1965, 13(4), 372-82,

[38] Franco, CB; et al., Distinguishing mast cell and granulocyte differentiation at the single-cell level. *Cell Stem Cell*, 2010, 6(4), 361-8,

[39] Tsai, M; et al., Induction of mast cell proliferation, maturation, and heparin synthesis by the rat c-kit ligand, stem cell factor. *Proc Natl Acad Sci U S A*, 1991, 88(14), 6382-6,

[40] Galli, SJ; Tsai, M; Wershil, BK. The c-kit receptor, stem cell factor, and mast cells. What each is teaching us about the others. *Am J Pathol*, 1993, 142(4), 965-74,

[41] Chabot, B; et al., The proto-oncogene c-kit encoding a transmembrane tyrosine kinase receptor maps to the mouse W locus. *Nature*, 1988, 335(6185), 88-9,

[42] Coussens, LM; Werb, Z. Inflammatory cells and cancer: think different! *J Exp Med*, 2001, 193(6), F23-6,

[43] Hanahan, D; Weinberg, RA. The hallmarks of cancer. *Cell*, 2000, 100(1), 57-70,

[44] Riccardi, VM. Cutaneous manifestation of neurofibromatosis: cellular interaction, pigmentation, and mast cells. *Birth Defects Orig Artic Ser*, 1981, 17(2), 129-45,

[45] Riccardi, VM. Mast-cell stabilization to decrease neurofibroma growth. Preliminary experience with ketotifen. *Arch Dermatol*, 1987, 123(8), 1011-6,

[46] Riccardi, VM. A controlled multiphase trial of ketotifen to minimize neurofibroma-associated pain and itching. *Arch Dermatol*, 1993, 129(5), 577-81,

[47] Brannan, CI; et al., Targeted disruption of the neurofibromatosis type-1 gene leads to developmental abnormalities in heart and various neural crest-derived tissues. *Genes Dev*, 1994, 8(9), 1019-29,

[48] Jacks, T; et al., Tumour predisposition in mice heterozygous for a targeted mutation in Nf1, *Nat Genet*, 1994, 7(3), 353-61,

[49] Cichowski, K; et al., Mouse models of tumor development in neurofibromatosis type 1, *Science*, 1999, 286(5447), 2172-6,

[50] Zhu, Y; et al., Neurofibromas in NF1: Schwann cell origin and role of tumor environment. *Science*, 2002, 296(5569), 920-2,

[51] Yang, FC; et al., Neurofibromin-deficient Schwann cells secrete a potent migratory stimulus for Nf1+/- mast cells. *J Clin Invest*, 2003, 112(12), 1851-61,

[52] Chen, S; et al., Nf1-/- Schwann cell-conditioned medium modulates mast cell degranulation by c-Kit-mediated hyperactivation of phosphatidylinositol 3-kinase. *Am J Pathol*, 2010, 177(6), 3125-32,

[53] McDaniel, AS; et al., Pak1 regulates multiple c-Kit mediated Ras-MAPK gain-in-function phenotypes in Nf1+/- mast cells. *Blood*, 2008, 112(12), 4646-54,

[54] Hiatt, K; et al., Loss of the nf1 tumor suppressor gene decreases fas antigen expression in myeloid cells. *Am J Pathol*, 2004, 164(4), 1471-9,

[55] Jaakkola, S; et al., Type 1 neurofibromatosis: selective expression of extracellular matrix genes by Schwann cells, perineurial cells, and fibroblasts in mixed cultures. *J Clin Invest*, 1989, 84(1), 253-61,

[56] Yang, FC; et al., Nf1+/- mast cells induce neurofibroma like phenotypes through secreted TGF-beta signaling. *Hum Mol Genet*, 2006, 15(16), 2421-37,

[57] Munchhof, AM; et al., Neurofibroma-associated growth factors activate a distinct signaling network to alter the function of neurofibromin-deficient endothelial cells. *Hum Mol Genet*, 2006, 15(11), 1858-69,

[58] Li, F; et al., Neurofibromin is a novel regulator of RAS-induced signals in primary vascular smooth muscle cells. *Hum Mol Genet*, 2006, 15(11), 1921-30,

[59] Yang, FC; et al., Nf1-dependent tumors require a microenvironment containing Nf1+/-- and c-kit-dependent bone marrow. *Cell*, 2008, 135(3), 437-48,

[60] Nocka, K; et al., Molecular bases of dominant negative and loss of function mutations at the murine c-kit/white spotting locus: W37, Wv, W41 and W. *EMBO J*, 1990, 9(6), 1805-13,

[61] Tan, JC; et al., The dominant W42 spotting phenotype results from a missense mutation in the c-kit receptor kinase. Science, 1990, 247(4939), 209-12,

[62] Zsebo, KM; et al., Stem cell factor is encoded at the Sl locus of the mouse and is the ligand for the c-kit tyrosine kinase receptor. *Cell*, 1990, 63(1), 213-24,

[63] Robertson, K.A., et al., Imatinib mesylate for plexiform neurofibromas in patients with neurofibromatosis type 1: a phase 2 trial. *Lancet Oncol*, 2012, 13(12), 1218-24,

INDEX

I

J

K